Clinical
Hematology
Atlas

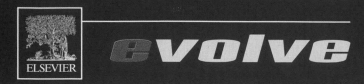

ELSEVIER

*:• *To access your Student Resources, visit:*

http://evolve.elsevier.com/Carr/hematology

Evolve® Student Resources for *Clinical Hematology Atlas,*
third edition, offer the following features:

- ## Summary Tables
  Tables showing images of cells together make it easier to compare and contrast cell morphology.

- ## Weblinks
  Links to places of interest on the Web specifically for hematology.

- ## Content Updates
  Find out the latest information on relevant issues in the field of hematology.

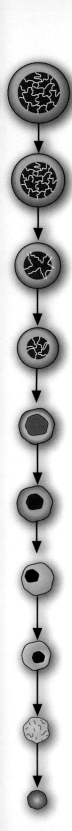

THIRD EDITION

Clinical
Hematology
Atlas

Jacqueline H. Carr, MS,
CLSpH(NCA), CLDir(NCA)
Laboratory Manager
Department of Pathology and Laboratory Medicine
Clarian Health
Indianapolis, Indiana

Bernadette F. Rodak, MS,
CLSpH(NCA)
Professor
Clinical Laboratory Science Program
Department of Pathology and Laboratory Medicine
Indiana University School of Medicine
Indianapolis, Indiana

SAUNDERS

ELSEVIER

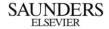

SAUNDERS
ELSEVIER

11830 Westline Industrial Drive
St. Louis, Missouri 63146

CLINICAL HEMATOLOGY ATLAS
Third Edition   ISBN 978-1-4160-5039-1
Copyright © 2009, 2004, 1999 by Saunders, an imprint of Elsevier Inc.

Notice

Library of Congress Control Number 2007938033

Publishing Director: Andrew Allen
Managing Editor: Ellen Wurm-Cutter
Publishing Services Manager: Patricia Tannian
Project Manager: Jonathan M. Taylor
Senior Designer: Amy Buxton

Printed in China.

Last digit is the print number: 9   8   7   6   5   4   3   2   1

To our husbands,
Robert Hartman
and
Charles Carr,
daughters,
Kimberly Carr Mayrose
and
Alexis Carr,
and all of the students
who have taught us hematology

Preface

Although there are several excellent hematology atlases available for use on personal computers and the Internet, in most instances this electronic medium does not lend itself well to morphologists who benefit by having photographs available when cells must be identified. Because the emphasis of an atlas is morphology, the *Clinical Hematology Atlas* is intended to be used with a textbook, such as Rodak BF, Fritsma GA, Doig K: *Hematology: Clinical Principles and Applications*, third edition, that addresses physiology and diagnosis along with morphology.

This atlas is designed for a diverse audience that includes clinical laboratory science students, medical students, residents, and practitioners. It is also a valuable resource for clinical laboratory practitioners who are being retrained or cross-trained in hematology.

Organization

As is frequently expounded, morphology on a peripheral blood film is only as good as the quality of the smear and the stain. Chapter 1 reviews smear preparation, staining, and the appropriate area in which to evaluate cell distribution and morphology. A table that summarizes the morphology of leukocytes found in a normal differential, along with multiple examples of each cell type, facilitates early instruction in blood smear review.

Chapter 2 schematically presents hematopoietic features of cell maturation. General cell maturation, along with an electron micrograph with labeled organelles, will help readers correlate the substructures with the appearance of cells under light microscopy. Visualizing normal cellular maturation is essential to the understanding of disease processes. This correlation of schematic, electron micrograph, and Wright-stained morphology is carried throughout the maturation chapters. Figure 2-1 has been reformatted to allow comparison of maturation stages across cell lines. In addition, the chart aids readers in recognizing the anatomical sites at which each stage of maturation normally occurs.

Chapters 3 to 9 present the maturation of each cell line individually, repeating the respective segment of the overall hematopoietic scheme from Chapter 2, to assist the student in seeing the relationship of each cell line to the whole. In these chapters, each maturation stage is presented as a color print, a schematic, and an electron micrograph. A description of each cell, including overall size, nuclear-to-cytoplasmic ratio, morphologic features, and reference ranges in peripheral blood and bone marrow, serves as a convenient summary. The final figure in each of these chapters summarizes lineage maturation by repeating the hematopoietic segment with the corresponding photomicrographs. New to this edition is the use of multiple nomenclatures for erythroid maturation, as well as the more common terminology for erythrocyte morphology.

Chapters 10 to 12 present discrete cellular abnormalities of erythrocytes, that is, variations in size, color, shape, and distribution, as well as inclusions found in erythrocytes. Each variation is presented along with a description of the abnormality, or composition of the inclusion, and associated disorders.

Because diseases are often combinations of the cellular alterations, Chapter 13 integrates morphologic findings into the diagnostic features of disorders primarily affecting erythrocytes.

In Chapters 14 and 15, nuclear and cytoplasmic alterations of leukocytes are displayed as a stepping stone to the correlations with leukocyte disorders.

Diseases of excessive or altered production of cells may be caused by maturation arrest, asynchronous development, or proliferation of one cell line, as presented in Chapters 15 to 20.

It is the authors' design that the cellular defects in leukocyte disorders be visually compared with the process of normal hematopoiesis for a more thorough comprehension of normal and altered development. Readers are encouraged to refer to the normal hematopoiesis illustration, Figure 2-1, for comparison of normal and abnormal cells and the progression of diseases. A new feature in this edition is the addition of a normal cell for comparison on the same page as a subtle alteration; for example, toxic granulation or agranulation compared with normal granulation.

Chapter 21 presents the most common stains, along with a summary chart for interpretation. Cytochemical stains aid in the diagnosis of leukoproliferative disorders. Microorganisms, including parasites, may be seen on peripheral blood smears. A brief photographic overview is given in Chapter 22. Additional organisms have been added, including *Ehrlichia* spp. and *Trypanosoma cruzi*. Readers are encouraged to consult a microbiology reference, such as Mahon CM, Lehman DC, Manuselis G: *Textbook of Diagnostic Microbiology*, third edition, for a more detailed presentation.

Chapter 23 includes photomicrographs that are not categorized into any one particular area, such as fat cells, mitotic figures, metastatic tumor cells, and artifacts.

Chapter 24 is new to the third edition and describes findings expected in the peripheral blood of neonates, including anticipated variations in morphology and cellular distribution.

Chapter 25 is intended to be an overview of the most frequent microscopic findings in body fluids. It is not proposed as a comprehensive review of the cytology of human body fluids, but rather a quick reference for the beginning microscopist as well as the seasoned professional.

The majority of the images for the third edition were taken using digital photography. The third edition also features spiral binding, making the atlas more convenient when used at the microscope bench.

All of these chapters combine into what we believe is a comprehensive and valuable resource for any clinical laboratory. The quality of the schematic illustrations, electron micrographs, and color photographs stand for themselves. We hope that this atlas will enrich the learning process for the student and serve as an important reference tool for the practitioner.

EVOLVE

New to the third edition is an Evolve website that provides free materials for both students and instructors. Instructors have access to an electronic image collection that features all of the images from the atlas. Students and instructors have access to summary tables, chapter quizzes, case studies, weblinks, and content updates.

Jacqueline H. Carr
Bernadette F. Rodak

Acknowledgments

From inception to completion we have had a great deal of assistance and encouragement from the faculty and staff of the Department of Pathology and Laboratory Medicine, Indiana University Medical Center. During the last two editions, the following individuals have "gone the extra mile" to help us continue to realize our dream. **Carol Bradford**, MT(ASCP)SH, Department of Medicine, for putting her extensive slide collection at our disposal; **George Girgis**, MT(ASCP), for sharing his incredible collection of body fluid slides, in addition to sharing his expertise in both blood cell and body fluid morphology; **Michael Goheen**, MS, Supervisor of the Electron Microscopy Laboratory, for his expertise and patience; **John Griep**, MD, Professor, Department of Pathology and Laboratory Medicine, Indiana University School of Medicine, for his expert advice and moral support; **Linda Marler** and **Jean Siders** for their technical assistance with digital photography and digital editing; **Linda Kasper** and **Linda Marler**, faculty members in the Clinical Laboratory Science program, for their support and patience during this endeavor. A particular thank you goes out to our families for their understanding during the many hours that we spent away from them while pursuing this goal.

A special thank you goes to the professionals at Elsevier who navigated us through the production of this atlas. **Ellen Wurm-Cutter**, Managing Editor, who has the patience of a saint and persevered with us, even when the going got rough; **Loren Wilson**, Executive Editor; **Jonathan Taylor**, Project Manager; and **Patricia Tannian**, Publishing Services Manager.

Contents

Clinical
Hematology
Atlas

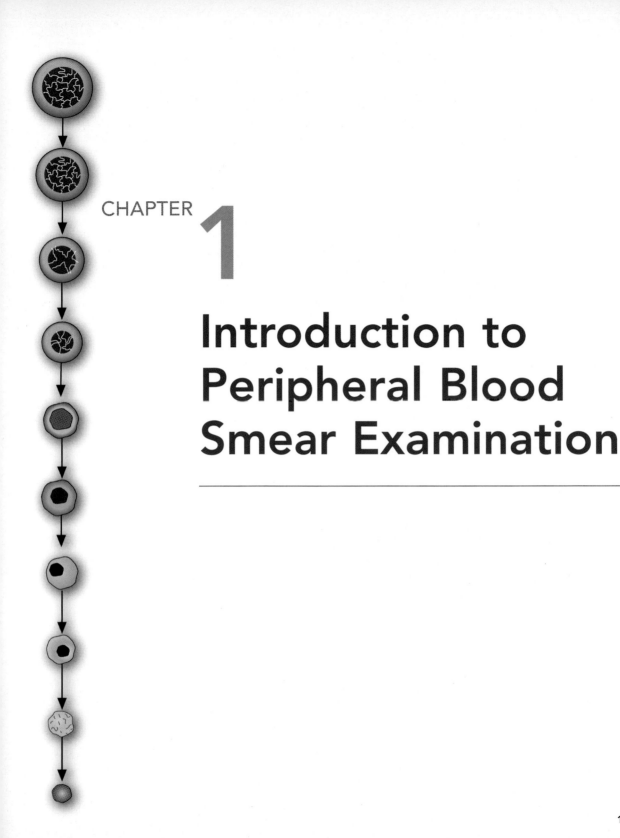

CHAPTER

1

Introduction to Peripheral Blood Smear Examination

A properly prepared blood smear is essential to accurate assessment of cellular morphology. A variety of methods are available for preparing and staining blood smears, the most common of which are discussed here. It is beyond the scope of this atlas to discuss other methodologies; however, detailed descriptions of these procedures can be found in a textbook of hematology.

WEDGE SMEAR PREPARATION

The wedge smear is the most convenient and commonly used technique for making peripheral blood smears. This technique necessitates at least two 3 × 1 inch (75 × 25 mm) clean glass slides. High-quality, beveled-edge microscope slides are recommended. One slide serves as the blood smear slide and the other as the spreader slide. These can then be reversed to prepare a second smear. A drop of ethylenediaminetetraacetic acid (EDTA) anticoagulated blood about 3 mm in diameter is placed at one end of the slide. Alternatively, a similar size drop of blood directly from a finger or heel puncture is acceptable. The size of the drop of blood is important. Too large a drop creates very long or thick smears, and too small a drop often makes a short or thin smear. In preparing the smear, the pusher slide is held securely in front of the drop of blood at a 30- to 45-degree angle to the smear slide (Figure 1-1, *A*). The pusher slide is pulled back into the drop of blood and held in that position until the blood spreads across the width of the slide (Figure 1-1, *B*). It is then quickly and smoothly pushed forward to the end of the smear slide, creating a wedge smear (Figure 1-1, *C*). It is important that the whole drop of blood is picked up and spread. Moving the pusher slide forward too slowly accentuates poor leukocyte distribution by pushing larger cells, such as monocytes and granulocytes, to the very end and sides of the smear. Maintaining a consistent angle between the slides and an even, gentle pressure is essential. It is frequently necessary to adjust the angle between the slides to produce a satisfactory smear. For higher-than-normal hematocrit, the angle between the slides must be lowered so that the smear is not too short and thick. For extremely low hematocrit, the angle must be raised. A well-made peripheral blood smear (Figure 1-2) has the following characteristics:

1. About two thirds to three fourths of the length of the slide is covered by the smear.
2. It is slightly rounded at featheredge (thin portion), not bullet shaped.
3. Lateral edges of the smear should be visible. The use of slides with chamfered (beveled) corners may facilitate this appearance.
4. It is smooth without irregularities, holes, or streaks.
5. When the slide is held up to light, the featheredge of the smear should have a "rainbow" appearance.
6. The whole drop is picked up and spread.

Figure 1-3 shows examples of unacceptable smears.

STAINING OF PERIPHERAL BLOOD SMEARS The purpose of staining blood smears is to identify cells and recognize morphology easily through the microscope. Wright stain or Wright-Giemsa stain is the most commonly used stain for peripheral blood and bone marrow smears. These contain both eosin and methylene blue and are therefore termed *polychrome stains.*

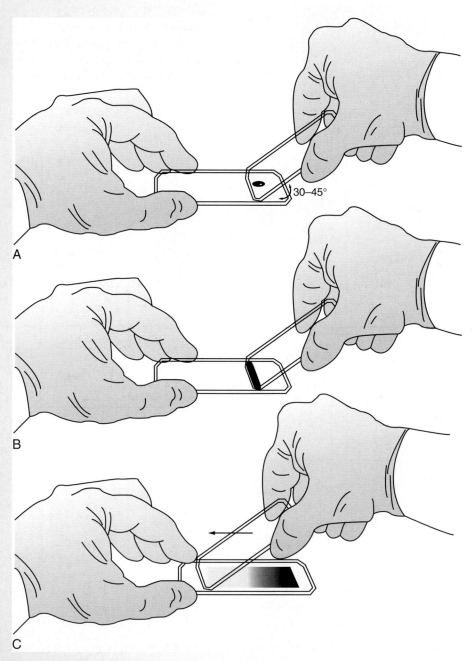

Figure 1-1 Wedge technique of making a peripheral blood smear. **A,** Correct angle to hold spreader slide. **B,** Blood spread across width of slide. **C,** Completed wedge smear. (From Rodak BF, Fritsma GA, Doig K: *Hematology: clinical principles and applications*, ed 3, Philadelphia, 2007, Saunders.)

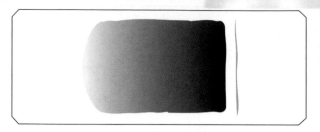

Figure 1-2 Well-made peripheral blood smear. (From Rodak BF, Fritsma GA, Doig K: *Hematology: clinical principles and applications,* ed 3, Philadelphia, 2007, Saunders.)

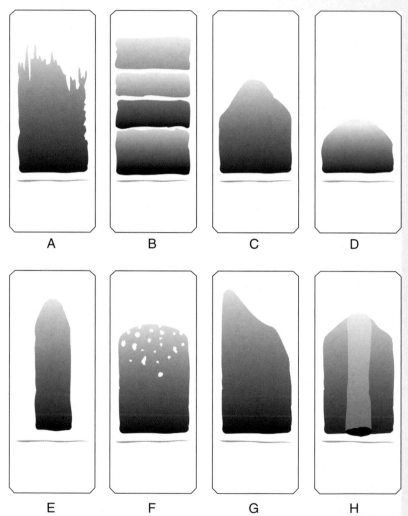

A

B

C

D

E

F

G

H

Figure 1-3 Examples of unacceptable smears and causes. **A,** Dirty slide. **B,** Skipping: uneven pressure during pushing. **C,** Improper angle of spreader slide; spreader slide movement too quick. **D,** Angle between slides is too large, or the drop of blood was too small (the opposite conditions result in a smear that is too long). **E,** Blood not allowed to spread across width of slide before smear was made. **F,** Hyperlipidemia, or oil on slide. **G,** Uneven pressure on sides of spreader slide. **H,** Drop of blood partially dried prior to pushing. (From Rodak BF, Fritsma GA, Doig K: *Hematology: clinical principles and applications,* ed 3, Philadelphia, 2007, Saunders.)

Figure 1-4 Optimally stained peripheral blood smear demonstrating the appropriate area in which to perform the white blood cell differential and morphology assessment and the platelet estimate. Only the center of the field is shown; an entire field would contain 200 to 250 red blood cells (×1000).

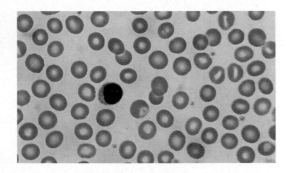

The cells are fixed to the glass slide by the methanol in the stain. Staining reactions are pH dependent, and the actual staining of the cellular components occurs when a buffer (pH 6.4) is added to the stain. Free methylene blue is basic and stains acidic cellular components, such as RNA, blue. Free eosin is acidic and stains basic components, such as hemoglobin or eosinophilic granules, red. Neutrophils have cytoplasmic granules that have a neutral pH and accept some characteristics from both stains. Details for specific methods of staining peripheral blood and bone marrow smears, including automated methods, may be found in a standard textbook of hematology.

An optimally stained smear (Figure 1-4) has the following characteristics:

1. The red blood cells (RBCs) should be pink to salmon in color.
2. Nuclei are dark blue to purple.
3. Cytoplasmic granules of neutrophils are lilac.
4. Cytoplasmic granules of basophils are dark blue to black.
5. Cytoplasmic granules of eosinophils are red to orange.
6. The area between the cells should be clean and free of precipitated stain.

A well-stained slide is necessary for accurate interpretation of cellular morphology. The best staining results are obtained from freshly made slides that have been prepared within 2 to 3 hours of blood collection. Slides must be allowed to dry thoroughly before staining. Box 1-1 lists common reasons for poorly stained slides and may be used as a guide when troubleshooting.

PERIPHERAL SMEAR EXAMINATION

10× EXAMINATION Examination of the blood smear is a multistep process. Begin the smear examination with a scan of the slide at 10× or low power. This step is necessary to assess the overall quality of the smear, including abnormal distribution of RBCs, suggesting the presence of rouleaux or autoagglutination and/or the presence of a disproportionate number of large nucleated cells, such as monocytes or neutrophils, at the edges of the smear. If the latter exists, another smear should be prepared. Additionally the 10× smear examination allows for the rapid detection of large abnormal cells such as blasts, reactive lymphocytes, and parasites.

40× EXAMINATION Using the 40× (high dry) objective, find an area of the smear in which the RBCs are evenly distributed and barely touching one another (two or three cells

> **BOX 1-1** Troubleshooting Poorly Stained Blood Smears
>
> **First Scenario**
> *Problems*
> - Red blood cells appear gray
> - White blood cells are too dark
> - Eosinophil granules are gray, not orange
>
> *Causes*
> - Stain or buffer too alkaline (most common)
> - Inadequate rinsing
> - Prolonged staining
> - Heparinized blood sample
>
> **Second Scenario**
> *Problems*
> - Red blood cells too pale or are red color
> - White blood cells barely visible
>
> *Causes*
> - Stain or buffer too acidic (most common)
> - Underbuffering (too short)
> - Overrinsing

From Rodak BF, Fritsma GA, Doig K: *Hematology: clinical principles and applications*, ed 3, Philadelphia, 2007, Saunders.

may overlap) (Figure 1-5). Scan 8 to 10 fields in this area of the smear and determine the average number of white blood cells (WBCs) per field. Multiply the average number of WBCs per high power field by 2000 to get an approximation of the total WBC count/mm^3. This estimate is a useful quality-control tool for validating WBC counts from hematology analyzers. Any discrepancy between the instrument WBC count and the slide estimate must be resolved. Some reasons for discrepancy are a mislabeled smear, a smear made from the wrong patient's sample, and an instrument malfunction.

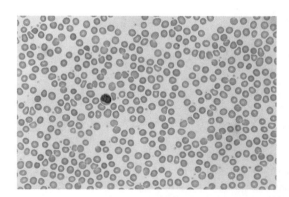

Figure 1-5 Correct area of blood smear in which to evaluate cellular distribution and perform WBC estimate (×400).

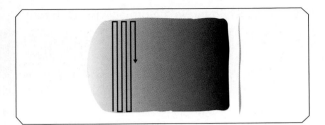

Figure 1-6 "Battlement" pattern for performing a white blood cell differential. (From Rodak BF, Fritsma GA, Doig K: *Hematology: clinical principles and applications,* ed 3, Philadelphia, 2007, Saunders.)

100× EXAMINATION. The next step in smear evaluation is to perform the WBC differential. This is done in the same area of the smear as the WBC estimate but using the 100× oil immersion objective. When the correct area of the smear from a patient with a normal RBC count is viewed, about 200 to 250 RBCs per oil immersion field are seen (see Figure 1-4). Characteristically the differential count includes counting and classifying 100 consecutive WBCs and reporting these classes as percentages. The differential count is performed in a systematic manner using the "battlement" track (Figure 1-6), which minimizes WBC distribution errors. The results are reported as percentages of each type of WBC seen during the count. An example of a WBC differential count is 3% bands, 55% polymorphonuclear neutrophils, 30% lymphocytes, 6% monocytes, 4% eosinophils, and 2% basophils (Table 1-1). Any WBC abnormalities, such as toxic changes, Döhle bodies, reactive lymphocytes, and Aüer rods, are also reported. When present, nucleated red blood cells (NRBCs) are counted and reported as number of NRBCs/100 WBCs. The RBC, WBC, platelet morphology evaluation, and the platelet estimates are also performed under the 100× oil immersion objective. RBC inclusions, such as Howell-Jolly bodies, and WBC inclusions, such as Döhle bodies, can be seen at this magnification. Each laboratory should have established protocols for standardized reporting of abnormalities.

Evaluation of the RBC morphology is an important aspect of the smear evaluation and is used in conjunction with the RBC indices to describe cells as normal or abnormal in size, shape, and color. Most laboratories use concise statements describing overall RBC morphology that is consistent with the RBC indices. The microscopic evaluation of RBC morphology must be congruent with the information given by the automated hematology analyzer. If not, discrepancies must be resolved before reporting patient results.

The final step in the performance of the differential count is the estimation of the platelet number. This is done under the 100× oil immersion objective. In an area of the smear where RBCs barely touch, the number of platelets in 10 oil immersion fields is counted. The average number of platelets is multiplied by 20,000 to provide an estimate of the total number of platelets present in the sample. This estimate is reported as adequate if the estimate is consistent with a normal platelet count, decreased if below the lower limit of normal for that laboratory, and increased if above the upper limit of normal. A general reference range is 150 to 450 × 10⁹/L (150,000 to 450,000/mm³). The estimate can be compared with an automated platelet count as an additional quality control measure.

It should be noted that high-quality, 40× or 50× oil immersion objectives can be used by the experienced technologist to perform the differential analysis of the blood smear. However, all abnormal findings must be verified under the 100× objective.

TABLE 1-1 Cells Found in a Normal WBC Differential

CELL TYPE	CELLS SIZE (μm)	NUCLEUS	CHROMATIN	CYTOPLASM	GRANULES	ADULT REFERENCE RANGE (PB) (%)	ADULT REFERENCE RANGE (Cells × 10⁹/L)
Polymorphonuclear neutrophil (Poly, PMN), segmented neutrophil (Seg)	10-15	2-5 lobes connected by thin filaments without visible chromatin	Coarsely clumped	Pale blue to pink	1°: Rare 2°: Abundant	50-70	2.3-8.1
Band Neutrophil (Band)	10-15	C or S shaped; constricted but no threadlike filament; chromatin must be visible in the filament	Coarsely clumped	Pale blue to pink	1°: Few 2°: Abundant	0-5	0.0-0.6
Lymphocyte (Lymph)	7-18*	Round to oval; may be slightly indented; occasional nucleoli	Condensed to deeply condensed	Scant to moderate; sky blue; vacuoles may be present	± Few azurophilic	20-40	0.8-4.8
Monocyte (Mono)	12-20	Variable; may be round, horse-shoe or kidney shaped. Often has folds producing "brainlike" convolutions	Lacy	Blue-gray; may have pseudopods; vacuoles may be absent or numerous	Many fine granules, frequently giving the appearance of ground glass	3-11	1.5-1.3
Eosinophil (Eos)	12-17	2-3 lobes connected by thin filaments without visible chromatin	Coarsely clumped	Pink; may have irregular borders	1°: Rare 2°: Abundant red to orange, round	0-5	0.0-0.4
Basophil (Baso)	10-14	Usually 2 lobes connected by thin filaments without visible chromatin	Coarsely clumped	Lavender to colorless	1°: Rare 2°: Variable in number with uneven distribution; may obscure nucleus or wash out during staining, giving the appearance of empty areas in cytoplasm	0-1	0.0-0.1

* The difference in size from small to large lymphocyte is due primarily to a larger amount of cytoplasm.

Microscopic View

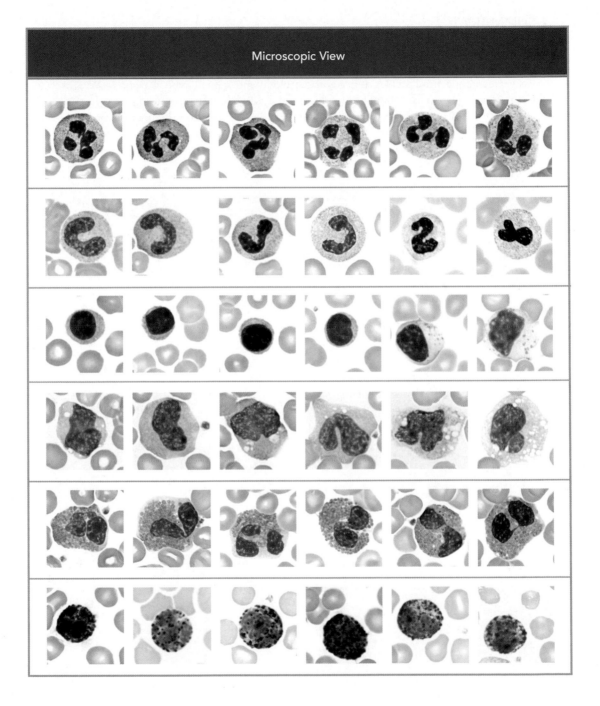

SUMMARY

A considerable amount of valuable information can be obtained from properly prepared, stained, and evaluated peripheral blood smears. Most laboratories use smears made by the wedge technique from EDTA anticoagulated blood and stained with Wright or Wright-Giemsa stain. The smears should be evaluated in a systematic manner using first the 10×, then 40× high dry, and finally the 100× oil immersion objectives on the microscope. White blood cell differential and morphology, and the RBC morphology and platelet estimate are included in the smear evaluation.

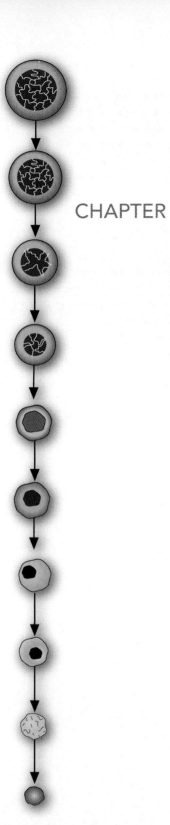

CHAPTER

2

Hematopoiesis

Hematopoiesis is a vigorous process of blood cell production and maturation that occurs primarily in the bone marrow. The process begins with the pluripotential stem cell, which is capable of proliferation, replication, and differentiation. In response to cytokines (growth factors), the pluripotential stem cell will differentiate into a myeloid or a lymphoid stem cell. Both the myeloid and lymphoid stem cells maintain their pluripotential capacity. The lymphoid stem cell differentiates into a committed pre-B or pre-T stem cell. The myeloid stem cell produces an intermediate stem cell, CFU–GEMM (colony forming unit–granulocyte, erythrocyte, monocyte, megakaryocyte) that in response to specific cytokines differentiates into erythroid, megakaryocytic, myeloid, monocytic, eosinophilic, or basophilic lineage. To this point in maturation, none of these stem cells can be morphologically identified, although it is postulated that they appear similar to a small resting lymphocyte. The blue shaded area in Figure 2-1 highlights the stem cell populations. Each lineage and maturation stage will be presented in detail in the following chapters.

Hematopoiesis is a dynamic continuum, that is, cells gradually mature from one stage to the next and may be between stages when viewed through the microscope. In general, the cell is then identified as the more mature stage. Figures 2-2 and 2-3 illustrate cell ultrastructure. A review of organelles will facilitate correlation of morphological maturation with cell function. This topic is explored in depth in hematology textbooks. Table 2-1 delineates the location, appearance, and function of individual organelles. General morphological changes in blood cell maturation (Figure 2-4) include the following:

- Basophilic cytoplasm to less basophilic
- Reduction in cell size
- Condensation of nuclear chromatin

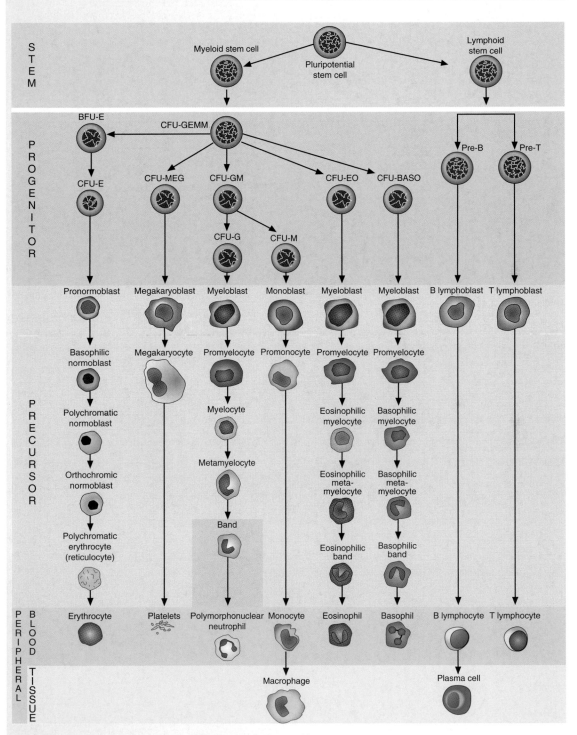

Figure 2-1 Chart of hematopoiesis.

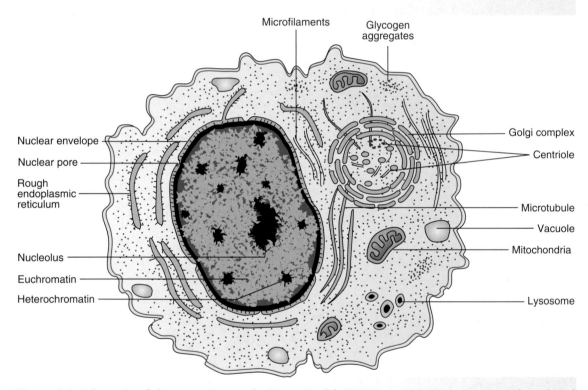

Figure 2-2 Schematic of electron micrograph. (From Rodak BF, Fritsma GA, Doig K: *Hematology: clinical principles and applications,* ed 3, Philadelphia, 2007, Saunders.)

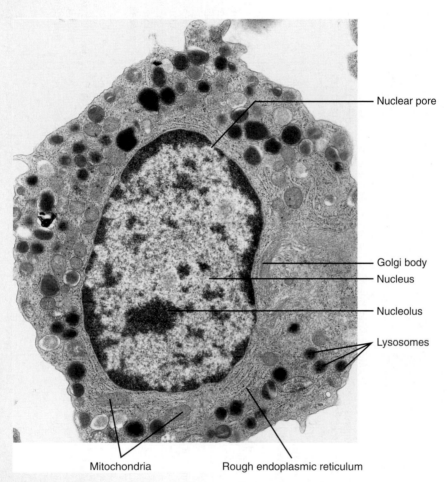

Nuclear pore

Golgi body
Nucleus
Nucleolus
Lysosomes

Mitochondria   Rough endoplasmic reticulum

Figure 2-3 Electron micrograph with labeled organelles.

TABLE 2-1 Summary of Cellular Components and Function

Organelle	Location	Appearance and Size by Electron Microscopy	Function	Comments
Membranes: nuclear, mitochondrial, endoplasmic reticulum	Outer boundary of cell, nucleus, endoplasmic reticulum, mitochondria, and other organelles	Usually a lipid bilayer consisting of proteins, cholesterol, phospholipids, and polysaccharides; membrane thickness varies with cell or organelle	Separates the plasma, various components; facilitates and restricts cellular exchange of substances	Membrane must be resilient and flexible
Nucleus	Within cell	Usually round or oval but varies depending on cell; varies in size; consists of DNA	The control center of the cell containing the genetic blueprint	Governs the cellular activity and transmits information for cellular control
Nucleolus	Within nucleus	Usually round or irregular in shape; 2-4 μm in size; composed of RNA; there may be 1-4 within nucleus	Site of synthesis and processing of various ribosomal RNA	Appearance varies with activity of the cells; larger when cell is actively involved in protein synthesis
Golgi body	Between nucleus and luminal surface of the cell	System of stacked membrane-bound flattened sacs; varies in size	Involved in modifying and packaging macromolecules for secretion	Well developed in cells with large secretion responsibilities
Endoplasmic reticulum	Randomly throughout cytoplasm	Membrane-lined tubules that branch and connect to nucleus and plasma membrane	Stores and transports fluids and chemicals	Two types: smooth with no ribosomes, rough with ribosomes on the surface

	Location	Structure	Function	Comments
Ribosomes	Free in cytoplasm; outer surface of rough endoplasmic reticulum	Small granule, 100-300 Å; composed of protein and nucleic acid	Protein production, such as enzymes and blood proteins	Large proteins are synthesized from polyribosomes (chains of ribosomes)
Mitochondria	Randomly in cytoplasm	Round or oval structures; 3-14 nm in length; 2-10 nm in width; membrane has 2 layers; inner layer has folds called cristae	Cell's "powerhouse"; makes ATP, the energy source for the cell	Active cells have more present than do inactive ones
Lysosomes	Randomly in cytoplasm	Membrane bound sacs; size varies	Contain hydrolytic enzymes for cellular digestive system	If the membrane breaks, the hydrolytic enzymes can destroy the cell
Microfilaments	Near nuclear envelope and within proximity of mitotic process	Small, solid structure approximately 5 nm in diameter	Support of cytoskeleton and motility	Consists of actin and myosin (contractile proteins)
Microtubules	Cytoskeleton, near nuclear envelope and component part of centriole near Golgi body	Hollow cylinder with protofilaments surrounding the outside tube; 20-25 nm in diameter, variable length	Maintenance of cell shape, motility, and the mitotic process	Produced from tubulin polymerization; make up mitotic spindles and part of the structure of the centriole
Centriole	In centrosome near nucleus	Cylinders; 150 nm in diameter, 300-500 nm in length	Serve as insertion points for mitotic spindle fibers	Nine sets of triplet microtubules

From Rodak BF, Fritsma GA, Doig K: *Hematology: clinical principles and applications*, ed 3, Philadelphia, 2007, Saunders.
ATP, Adenosine triphosphate.

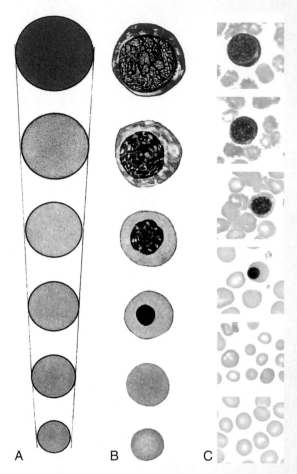

A   B   C

Figure 2-4 A, General cellular maturation: changes in cell size and color. **B,** General cell maturation: changes in nuclear size and chromatin condensation. NOTE: Red blood cell loses nucleus. White blood cell nucleus is retained and undergoes further maturation. **C,** Representative cells. (From Diggs LW, Sturm D, and Bell A: *The morphology of human blood cells*, ed 5, Abbott Park, Ill, 1985, Abbott Laboratories. Reproduction of *The Morphology of Human Blood Cells* has been granted with approval of Abbott Laboratories, all rights reserved by Abbott Laboratories.)

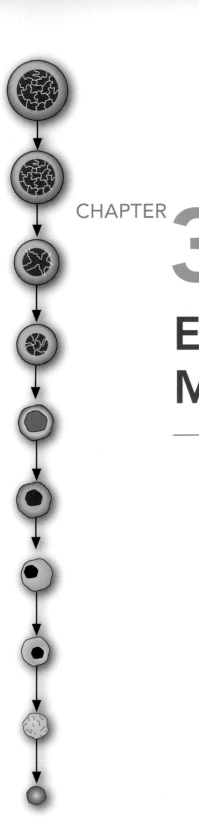

3

Erythroid Maturation

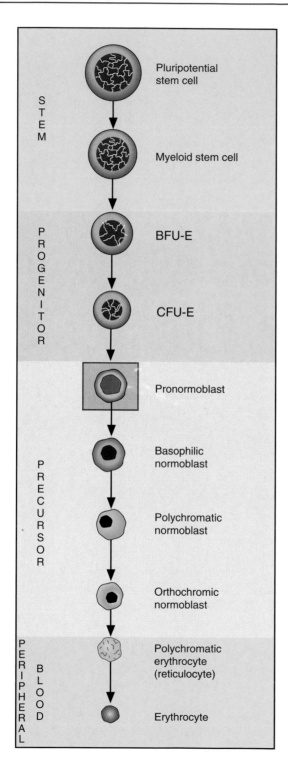

Figure 3-1 Erythroid sequence–Pronormoblast.

PRONORMOBLAST
Proerythroblast
Rubriblast

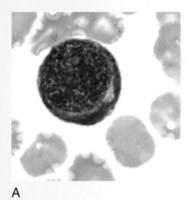

A

Figure 3-2A Pronormoblast.

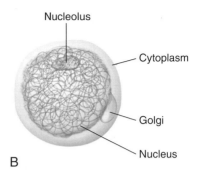

B

Figure 3-2B Schematic of pronormoblast.

SIZE: 12-20 μm
NUCLEUS: Round
Nucleoli: 1-2
Chromatin: Fine
CYTOPLASM: Dark blue
N/C RATIO: 8:1
REFERENCE INTERVAL:
Bone Marrow: 1%
Peripheral Blood: 0%

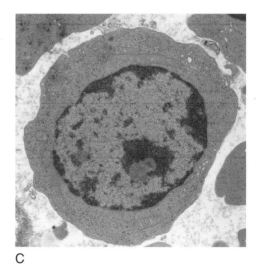

C

Figure 3-2C Electron micrograph of pronormoblast (×15,575).

All photomicrographs are ×1000 with Wright–Giemsa stain unless stated otherwise.

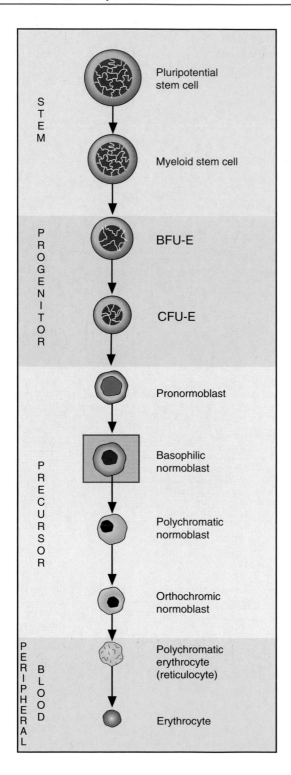

Figure 3-3 Erythroid sequence–Basophilic normoblast.

BASOPHILIC NORMOBLAST
Basophilic Erythroblast
Prorubricyte

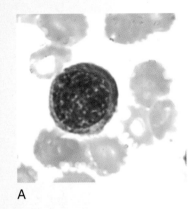

A

Figure 3-4A Basophilic normoblast.

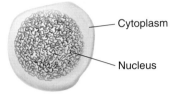

Cytoplasm

Nucleus

B

Figure 3-4B Schematic of basophilic normoblast.

SIZE: 10-15 μm
NUCLEUS: Round
Nucleoli: 0-1
Chromatin: Slightly condensed
CYTOPLASM: Dark blue
N/C RATIO: 6:1
REFERENCE INTERVAL:
Bone Marrow: 1%-4%
Peripheral Blood: 0%

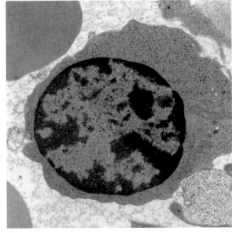

C

Figure 3-4C Electron micrograph of basophilic normoblast (×15,575).

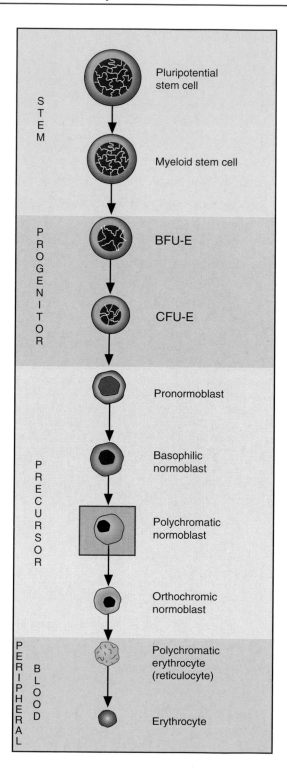

Figure 3-5 Erythroid sequence—Polychromatic normoblast.

POLYCHROMATIC NORMOBLAST
Polychromatic Erythroblast
Rubricyte

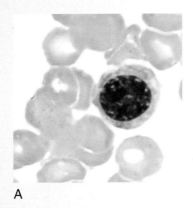

A

Figure 3-6A Polychromatic normoblast.

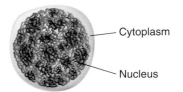

Cytoplasm

Nucleus

B

Figure 3-6B Schematic of polychromatic normoblast.

SIZE: 10-12 μm
NUCLEUS: Round
Nucleoli: 0
Chromatin: Quite condensed
CYTOPLASM: Gray blue
N/C RATIO: 4:1
REFERENCE INTERVAL:
Bone Marrow: 10%-20%
Peripheral Blood: 0%

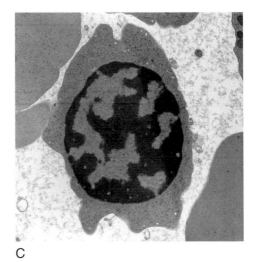

C

Figure 3-6C Electron micrograph of polychromatic normoblast (×15,575).

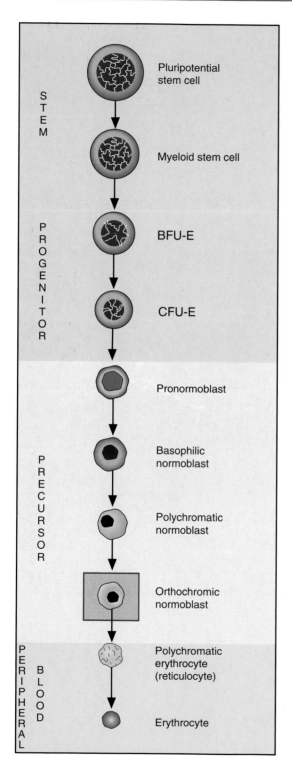

Figure 3-7 Erythroid sequence–Orthochromic normoblast.

ORTHOCHROMIC NORMOBLAST
Orthochromic Erythroblast
Metarubricyte

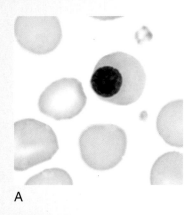

A

Figure 3-8A Orthochromic normoblast.

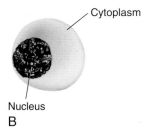

Cytoplasm

Nucleus

B

Figure 3-8B Schematic of orthochromic normoblast.

SIZE: 8-10 μm
NUCLEUS: Round
Nucleoli: 0
Chromatin: Fully condensed
CYTOPLASM: Blue to salmon
N/C RATIO: 0.5:1
REFERENCE INTERVAL:
Bone Marrow: 5%-10%
Peripheral Blood: 0%

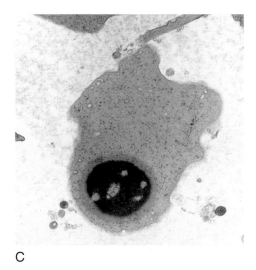

C

Figure 3-8C Electron micrograph of orthochromic normoblast (×20,125).

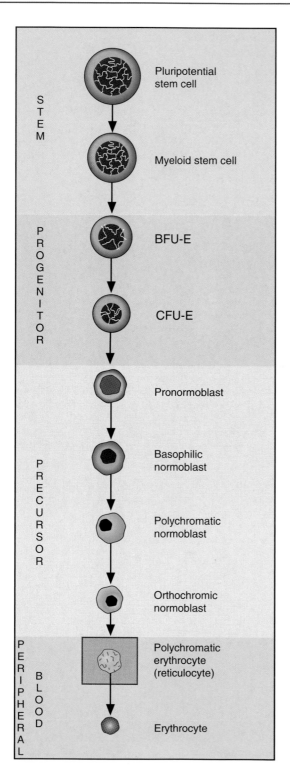

Figure 3-9 Erythroid sequence–Polychromatic erythrocyte (reticulocyte).

POLYCHROMATIC ERYTHROCYTE
Diffusely Basophilic Erythrocyte
Reticulocyte

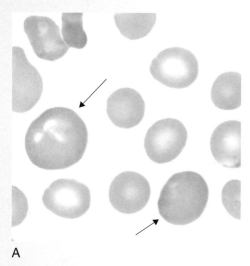

A

Figure 3-10A Polychromatic erythrocyte.

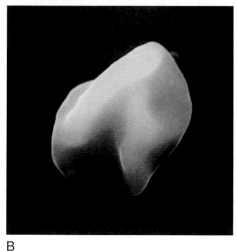

B

Figure 3-10B Scanning electron micrograph of polychromatic erythrocyte (×5000).

SIZE: 8-8.5 μm
NUCLEUS: Absent
Nucleoli: NA
Chromatin: NA
CYTOPLASM: Blue to salmon
N/C RATIO: NA
REFERENCE INTERVAL:
Bone Marrow: 1%
Peripheral Blood: 0.5%-2.0%
NOTE: When stained with supravital stain (e.g., new methylene blue), polychromatic erythrocytes appear as reticulocytes.

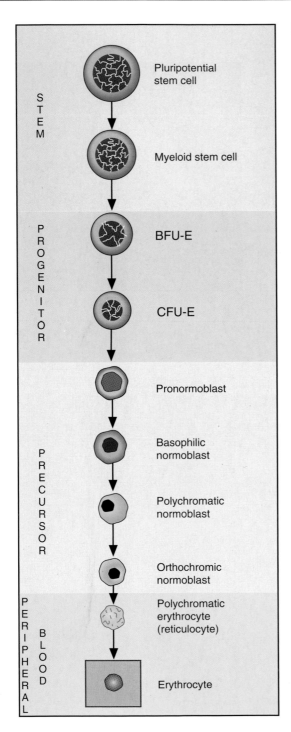

Figure 3-11 Erythroid Sequence—Erythrocyte.

ERYTHROCYTE

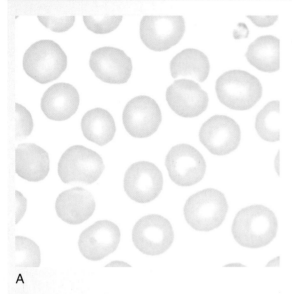

A

Figure 3-12A Erythrocyte.

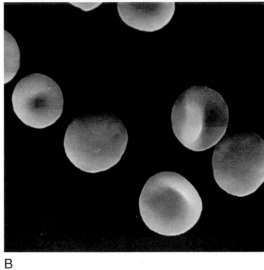

B

Figure 3-12B Scanning electron micrograph of erythrocyte (×2500).

SIZE: 7-8 μm
NUCLEUS: Absent
Nucleoli: NA
Chromatin: NA
CYTOPLASM: Salmon
N/C RATIO: NA
REFERENCE INTERVAL:
Bone Marrow: NA
Peripheral Blood: Predominant cell type

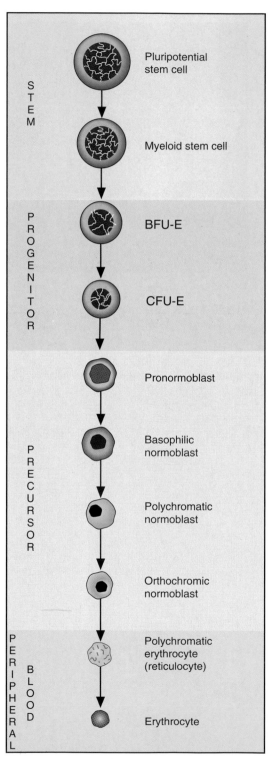

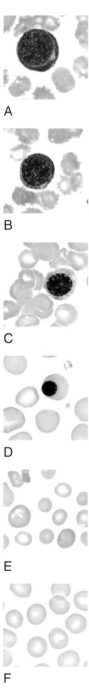

Figure 3-13 Erythrocyte sequence with **(A)** pronormoblast, **(B)** basophilic normoblast, **(C)** polychromatic normoblast, **(D)** orthochromic normoblast, **(E)** polychromatic erythrocyte, and **(F)** erythrocyte.

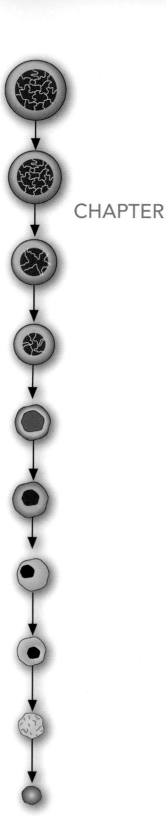

CHAPTER

4

Megakaryocyte
Maturation

Figure 4-1 Megakaryocytic sequence–
Megakaryocyte.

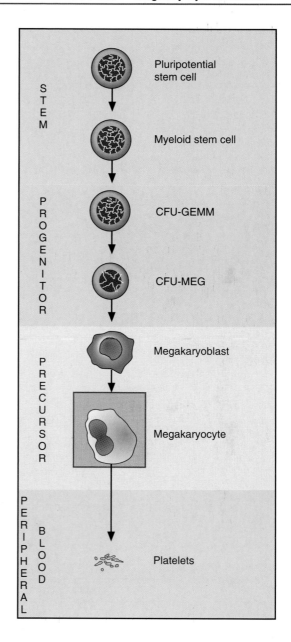

Megakaryoblasts cannot be identified with certainty by Wright–Giemsa stain. All photomicrographs are ×1000 with Wright–Giemsa stain unless stated otherwise.

MEGAKARYOCYTE

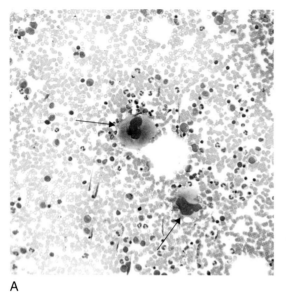

A

Figure 4-2A Megakaryocyte, early stage–Bone marrow (×100).

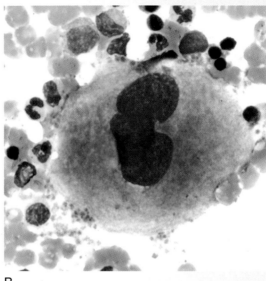

B

Figure 4-2B Megakaryocyte, early stage–Bone marrow (×500).

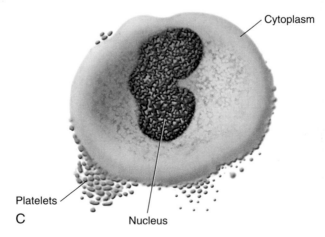

C

Figure 4-2C Schematic of megakaryocyte.

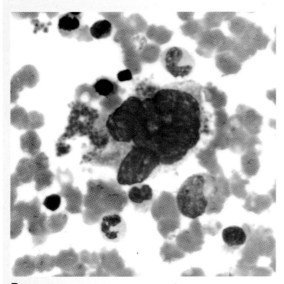

D

Figure 4-2D Megakaryocyte, late stage—Bone marrow (×500).

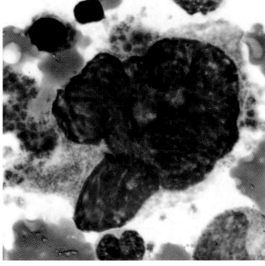

E

Figure 4-2E Megakaryocyte, late stage—Bone marrow (×1000).

SIZE: 20-90 μm
NUCLEUS: 2-16 lobes (8 lobes: most common)
NOTE: The size of the cell varies according to number of lobes present.
CYTOPLASM: Blue to pink; abundant
Granules: Reddish blue; few to abundant
N/C RATIO: Variable
REFERENCE INTERVAL:
Bone Marrow: 5-10 per 10× objective (100× magnification)
    1-2 per 50× objective (500× magnification)
NOTE: Megakaryocytes are usually reported as adequate, increased, or decreased and not as a percentage.
Peripheral Blood: 0%

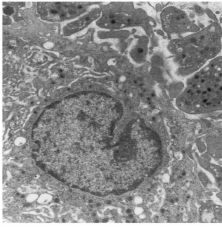

F

Figure 4-2F Electron micrograph of megakaryocyte (×16,500).

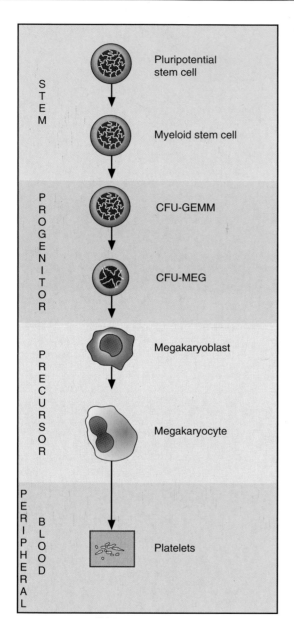

Figure 4-3 Megakaryocytic sequence–Platelets.

PLATELET

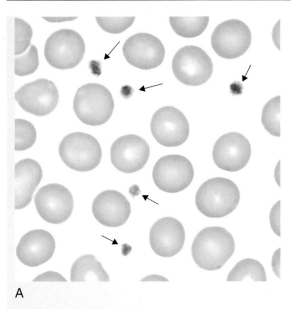

A

Figure 4-4A Platelet.

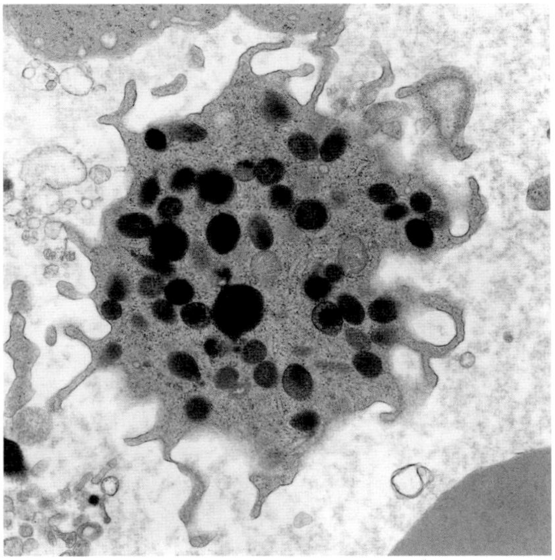

B

Figure 4-4B Electron micrograph of platelet (×28,750).

SIZE: 2-4 μm
NUCLEUS: NA
CYTOPLASM: Light blue to colorless
Granules: Red to violet
N/C RATIO: NA
REFERENCE INTERVAL:
Bone Marrow: NA
Peripheral Blood: 7-25 per 100× oil immersion field

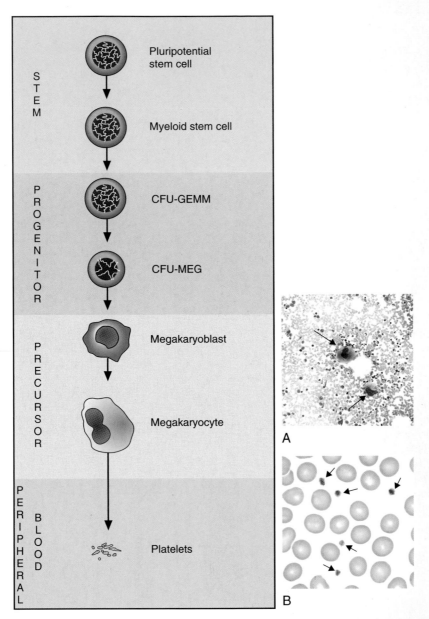

Figure 4-5 Megakaryocytic sequence with **(A)** megakaryocyte and **(B)** platelet.

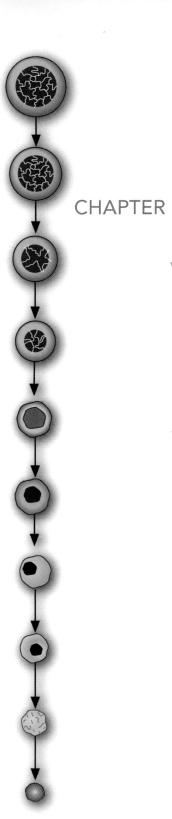

CHAPTER

5

Myeloid Maturation

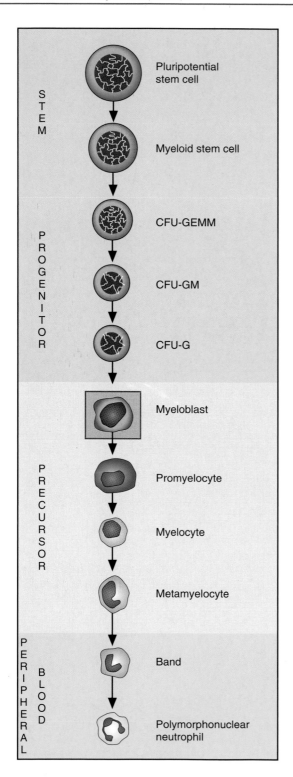

Figure 5-1 Myeloid sequence—Myeloblast.

MYELOBLAST

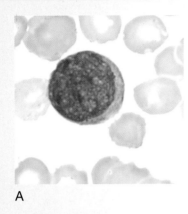

A

Figure 5-2A Myeloblast.

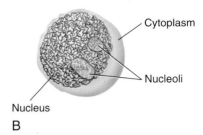

Cytoplasm

Nucleoli

Nucleus

B

Figure 5-2B Schematic of myeloblast.

SIZE: 15-20 µm
NUCLEUS: Round to oval
Nucleoli: 2-5
Chromatin: Fine
CYTOPLASM: Moderate basophilia
Granules: Absent or rare
N/C RATIO: 4:1
REFERENCE INTERVAL:
Bone Marrow: 0%-1%
Peripheral Blood: 0%

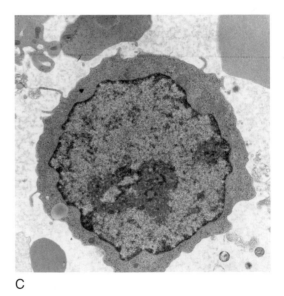

C

Figure 5-2C Electron micrograph of myeloblast (×16,500).

All photomicrographs are ×1000 with Wright–Giemsa stain unless stated otherwise.

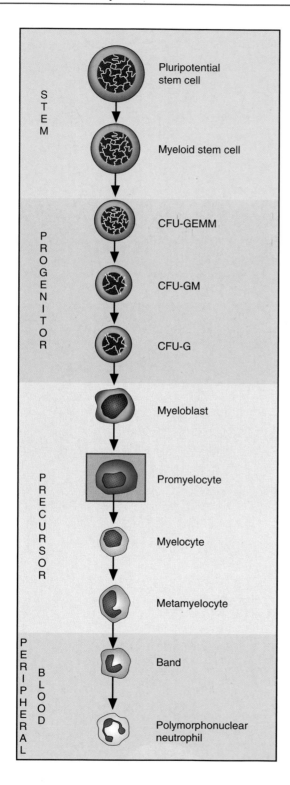

Figure 5-3 Myeloid sequence—Promyelocyte.

PROMYELOCYTE

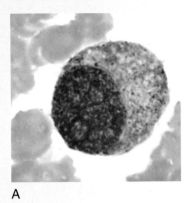

A

Figure 5-4A Promyelocyte.

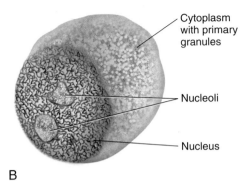

Cytoplasm
with primary
granules

Nucleoli

Nucleus

B

Figure 5-4B Schematic of promyelocyte.

SIZE: 14-20 μm
NUCLEUS: Round to oval
Nucleoli: 1-3 or more
Chromatin: Slightly coarser than myeloblast
CYTOPLASM: Basophilic
Granules:
   Primary: Few to many, red to purple
   Secondary: None
N/C RATIO: 3:1
REFERENCE INTERVAL:
Bone Marrow: 2%-5%
Peripheral Blood: 0%

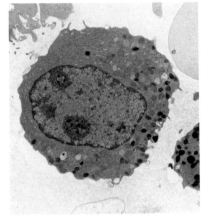

C

Figure 5-4C Electron micrograph of
promyelocyte (×13,000).

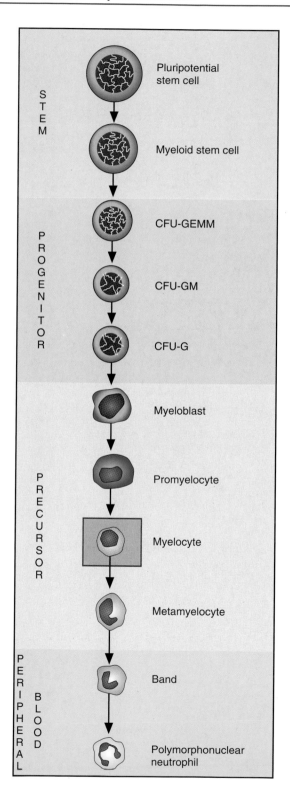

Figure 5-5 Myeloid sequence—Myelocyte.

MYELOCYTE

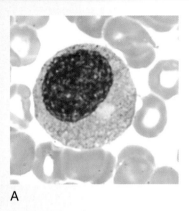

Figure 5-6A Myelocyte.

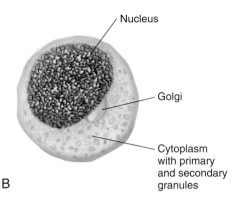

Nucleus

Golgi

Cytoplasm
with primary
and secondary
granules

B

Figure 5-6B Schematic of myelocyte.

SIZE: 12-18 μm

NUCLEUS: Round to oval; may have one
flattened side

Nucleoli: Usually not visible

Chromatin: Coarse and more condensed than
promyelocyte

CYTOPLASM: Slightly basophilic

Granules:
   Primary: Few to moderate
   Secondary: Variable number

N/C RATIO: 2:1

REFERENCE INTERVAL:

Bone Marrow: 5%-19%

Peripheral Blood: 0%

NOTE: As the cell matures, secondary
granules differentiate the cell lineage into
neutrophil, eosinophil, or basophil.

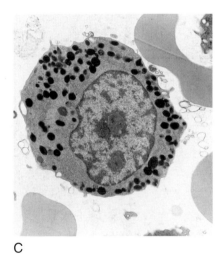

C

Figure 5-6C Electron micrograph of myelocyte
(×16,500).

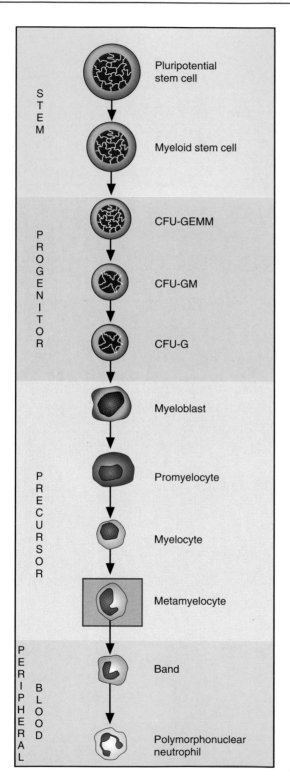

Figure 5-7 Myeloid sequence—Metamyelocyte.

METAMYELOCYTE

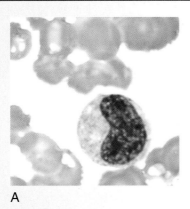

A

Figure 5-8A Metamyelocyte.

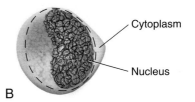

B

Figure 5-8B Schematic of metamyelocyte.
Dotted line indicates hypothetical round nucleus.

SIZE: 10-15 μm
NUCLEUS: Indented; kidney bean shape.
   Indentation is less than 50% of the width of
   a hypothetical round nucleus.
Nucleoli: Not visible
Chromatin: Coarse clumped
CYTOPLASM: Pale blue to pink
Granules:
   Primary: Few
   Secondary: Many (full complement)
N/C RATIO: 1.5:1
REFERENCE INTERVAL:
Bone Marrow: 13%-22%
Peripheral Blood: 0%

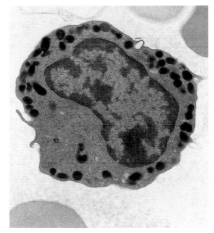

C

Figure 5-8C Electron micrograph of
metamyelocyte (×22,250).

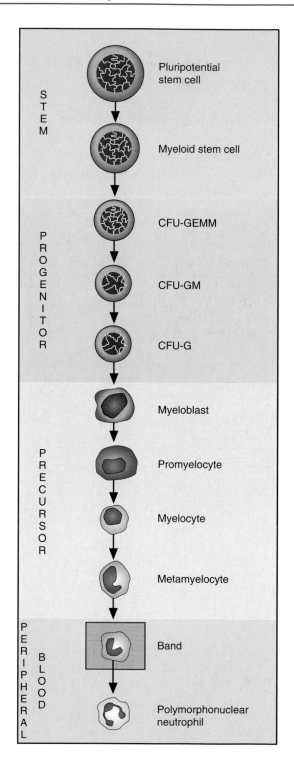

Figure 5-9 Myeloid sequence—Band.

BAND

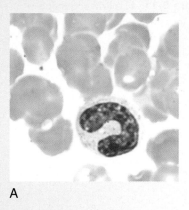

A

Figure 5-10A Band.

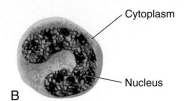

Cytoplasm

Nucleus

B

Figure 5-10B Schematic of band.

SIZE: 10-15 μm
NUCLEUS: C or S shaped. Constricted but no threadlike filament.
NOTE: Chromatin must be visible in constriction. May be folded over.
Nucleoli: Not visible
Chromatin: Coarse clumped
CYTOPLASM: Pale blue to pink
Granules:
   Primary: Few
   Secondary: Abundant
N/C RATIO: Cytoplasm predominates
REFERENCE INTERVAL:
Bone Marrow: 17%-33%
Peripheral Blood: 0%-5%
Refer to Table 1-1 for more examples.

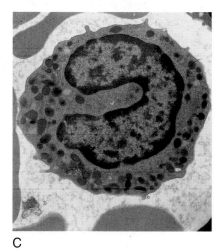

C

Figure 5-10C Electron micrograph of band (×22,250).

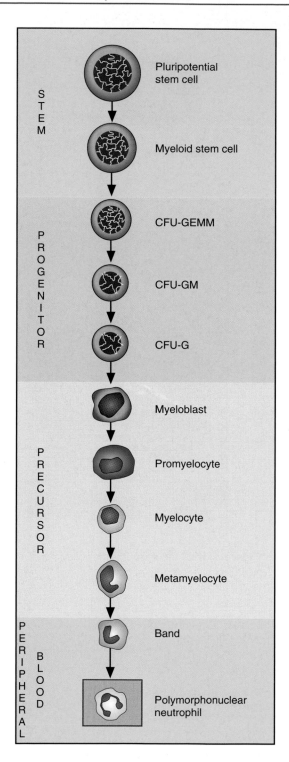

Figure 5-11 Myeloid sequence—Polymorphonuclear neutrophil.

POLYMORPHONUCLEAR NEUTROPHIL (PMN)

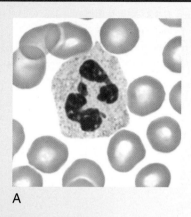

A

Figure 5-12A Polymorphonuclear neutrophil.

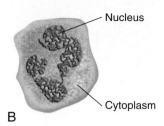

B

Figure 5-12B Schematic of polymorphonuclear neutrophil.

SIZE: 10-15 μm
NUCLEUS: 2-5 lobes connected by thin filaments without visible chromatin
Nucleoli: Not visible
Chromatin: Coarse clumped
CYTOPLASM: Pale blue to pink
Granules:
    Primary: Rare
    Secondary: Abundant
N/C RATIO: Cytoplasm predominates
REFERENCE INTERVAL:
Bone Marrow: 3%-11%
Peripheral Blood: 50%-70%

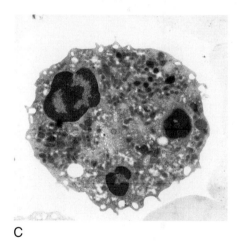

C

Figure 5-12C Electron micrograph of polymorphonuclear neutrophil (×22,250).

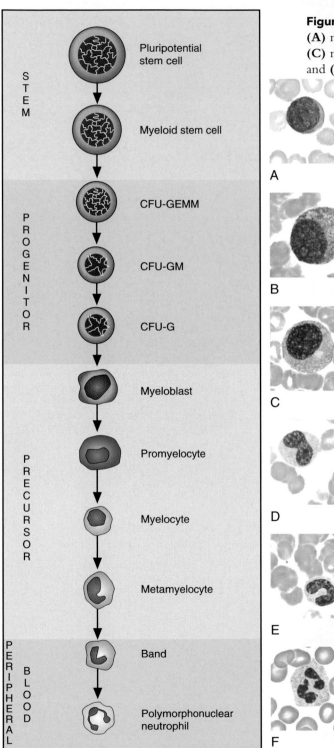

Figure 5-13 Myeloid sequence with **(A)** myeloblast, **(B)** promyelocyte, **(C)** myelocyte, **(D)** metamyelocyte, **(E)** band, and **(F)** polymorphonuclear neutrophil.

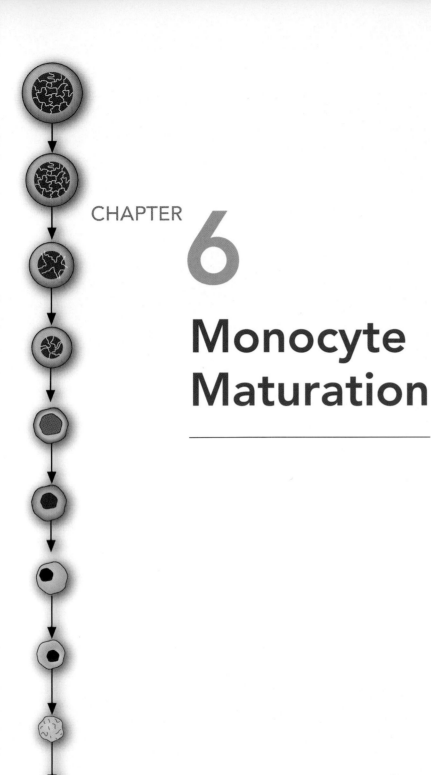

CHAPTER

6

Monocyte Maturation

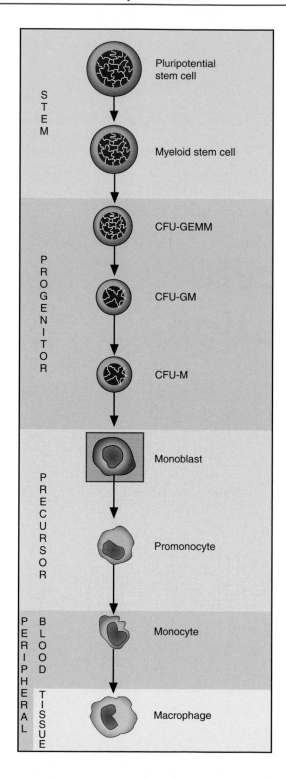

Figure 6-1 Monocyte sequence—Monoblast.

MONOBLAST

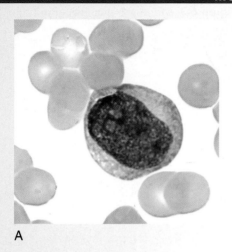

A

Figure 6-2A Monoblast.

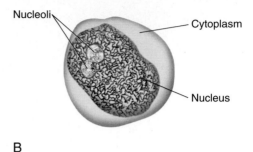

B

Figure 6-2B Schematic of monoblast.

SIZE: 12-18 μm
NUCLEUS: Round to oval; eccentric
Nucleoli: 1-2; may not be visible
Chromatin: Fine
CYTOPLASM: Deeply basophilic; may have a grayish tint
Granules: None
N/C RATIO: 4:1
REFERENCE INTERVAL:
Bone Marrow: Not defined
Peripheral Blood: None

All photomicrographs are ×1000 with Wright–Giemsa stain unless stated otherwise.

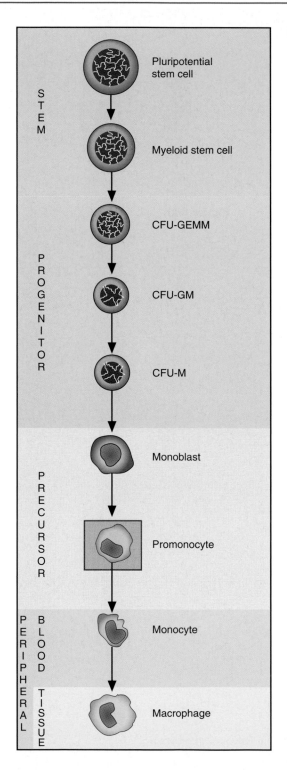

Figure 6-3 Monocyte sequence—Promonocyte.

PROMONOCYTE

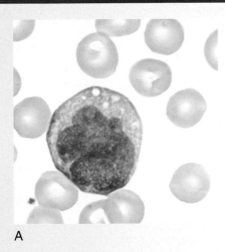

A

Figure 6-4A Promonocyte.

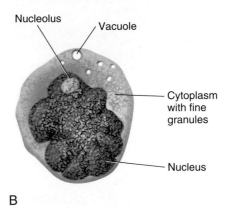

B

Figure 6-4B Schematic of promonocyte.

SIZE: 12-20 μm
NUCLEUS: Irregularly shaped; deeply indented
Nucleoli: May or may not be visible
Chromatin: Fine
CYTOPLASM: Blue to gray
Granules: Fine azurophilic
N/C RATIO: 2-3:1
REFERENCE INTERVAL:
Bone Marrow: <1%
Peripheral Blood: 0%

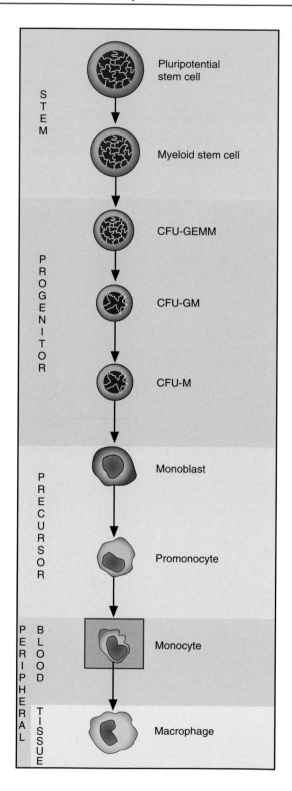

Figure 6-5 Monocyte sequence—Monocyte.

MONOCYTE

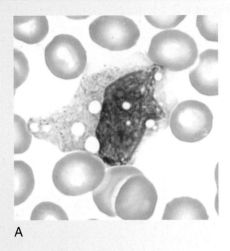

A

Figure 6-6A Monocyte.

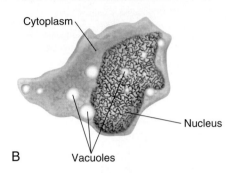

B

Figure 6-6B Schematic of monocyte.

SIZE: 12-20 μm
NUCLEUS: Variable; may be round, horseshoe-shaped or kidney-shaped. Often has folds producing "brainlike" convolutions.
Nucleoli: Not visible
Chromatin: Lacy
CYTOPLASM: Blue-gray; may have pseudopods
Granules: Many fine granules frequently giving the appearance of ground glass
Vacuoles: Absent to numerous
N/C RATIO: Variable
REFERENCE INTERVAL:
Bone Marrow: 2%
Peripheral Blood: 3%-11%

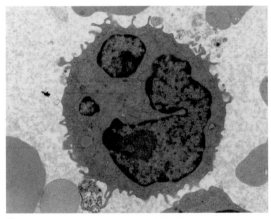

C

Figure 6-6C Electron micrograph of monocyte (×16,500).

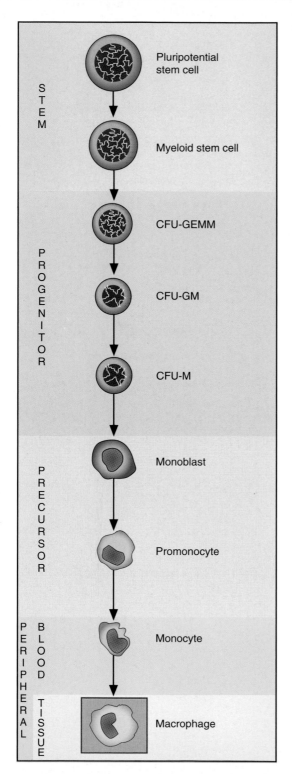

Figure 6-7 Monocyte sequence—Macrophage.

MACROPHAGE

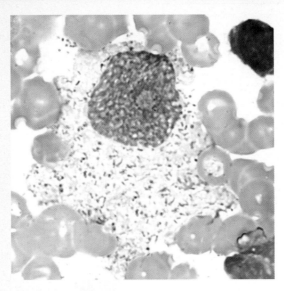

Figure 6-8 Macrophage.

SIZE: 15-80 μm
NUCLEUS: Eccentric, reniform, egg-shaped, indented, or elongated
Nucleoli: 1-2
Chromatin: Fine, dispersed
CYTOPLASM: Abundant with irregular borders; may contain ingested material
Granules: Many coarse azurophilic
Vacuoles: May be present
REFERENCE INTERVAL: NA
Refer to Table 1-1 for more examples.

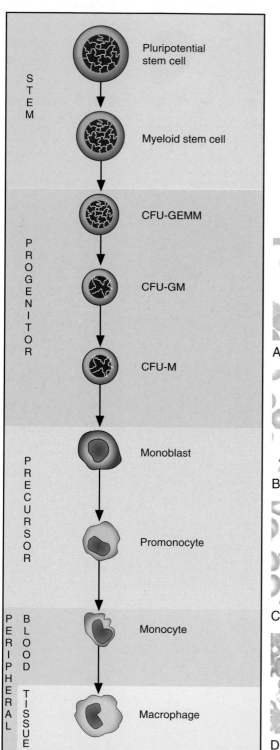

STEM

- Pluripotential stem cell
- Myeloid stem cell

PROGENITOR

- CFU-GEMM
- CFU-GM
- CFU-M

PRECURSOR

- Monoblast
- Promonocyte

PERIPHERAL BLOOD

- Monocyte

TISSUE

- Macrophage

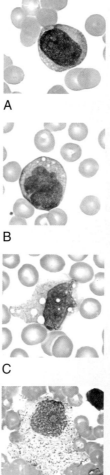

A

B

C

D

Figure 6-9 Monocyte sequence with **(A)** monoblast, **(B)** promonocyte, **(C)** monocyte, and **(D)** macrophage.

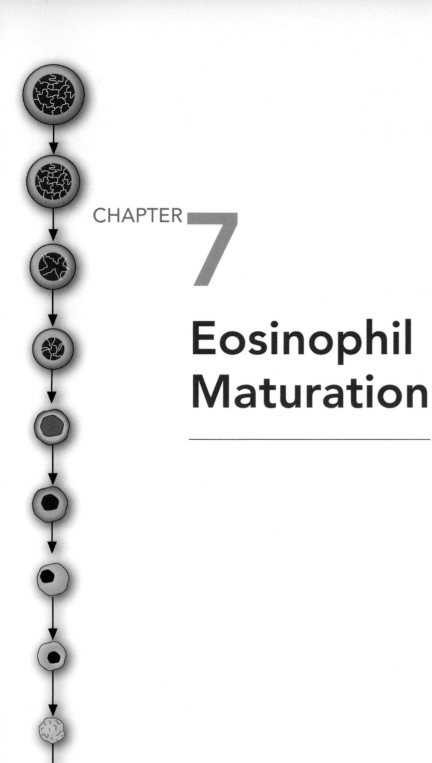

CHAPTER

7

Eosinophil Maturation

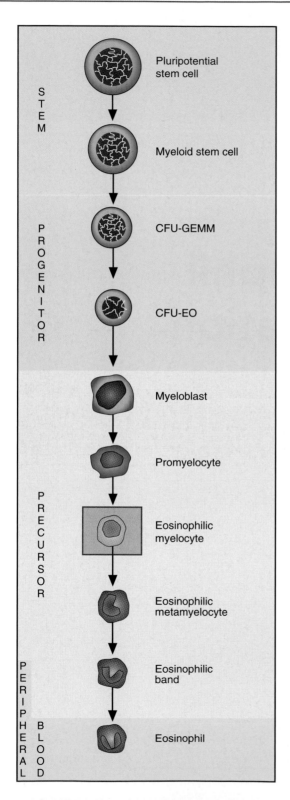

Figure 7-1 Eosinophilic sequence—Eosinophilic myelocyte.

EOSINOPHILIC MYELOCYTE

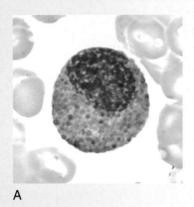

A

Figure 7-2A Eosinophilic myelocyte.

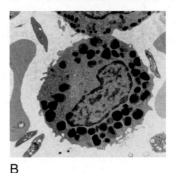

B

Figure 7-2B Electron micrograph of eosinophilic myelocyte.

SIZE: 12-18μm
NUCLEUS: Round to oval; may have one flattened side
Nucleoli: Usually not visible
Chromatin: Coarse and more condensed than promyelocyte
CYTOPLASM: Colorless to pink
Granules:
  Primary: Few to moderate
  Secondary: Variable number; orange to red; round
N/C RATIO: 2:1
REFERENCE INTERVAL:
Bone Marrow: 0%-2%
Peripheral Blood: 0%

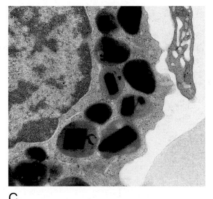

C

Figure 7-2C Electron micrograph of eosinophilic granule to demonstrate internal structures.

All photomicrographs are ×1000 with Wright-Giemsa stain unless stated otherwise.

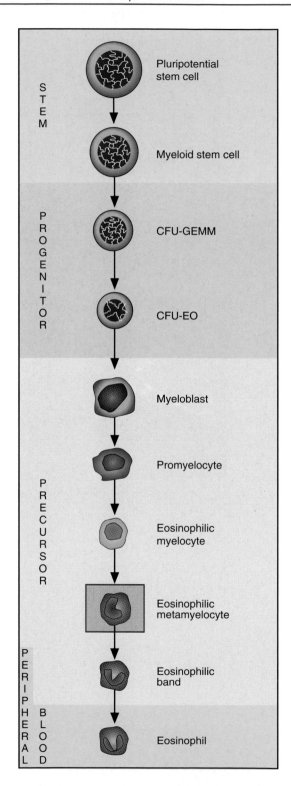

Figure 7-3 Eosinophilic sequence—Eosinophilic metamyelocyte.

EOSINOPHILIC METAMYELOCYTE

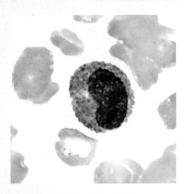

Figure 7-4 Eosinophilic metamyelocyte.

SIZE: 10-15 µm
NUCLEUS: Indented
Nucleoli: Not visible
Chromatin: Coarse clumped
CYTOPLASM: Colorless to pink
Granules:
   Primary: Few
   Secondary: Many red to orange; round
N/C RATIO: 1.5:1
REFERENCE INTERVAL:
Bone Marrow: 0%-2%
Peripheral Blood: 0%

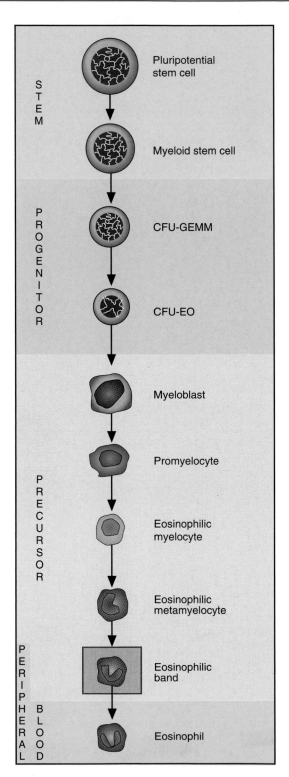

Figure 7-5 Eosinophilic sequence— Eosinophilic band.

EOSINOPHILIC BAND

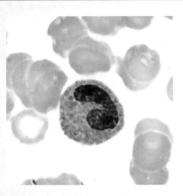

Figure 7-6 Eosinophilic band.

SIZE: 10-15 μm
NUCLEUS: Band-shaped. Constricted but no threadlike filament.
NOTE: Chromatin must be visible in constriction.
Nucleoli: Not visible
Chromatin: Coarse clumped
CYTOPLASM: Colorless to pink
Granules:
  Primary: Few
  Secondary: Abundant red to orange; round
N/C RATIO: Cytoplasm predominates
REFERENCE INTERVAL:
Bone Marrow: 0%-2%
Peripheral Blood: Rarely seen

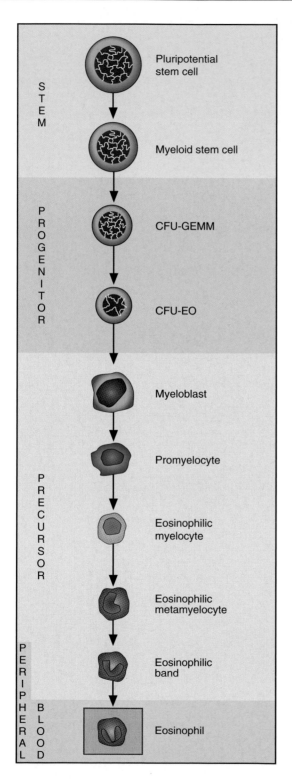

Figure 7-7 Eosinophilic sequence—Eosinophil.

EOSINOPHIL

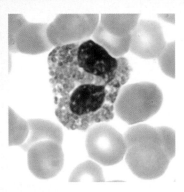

Figure 7-8 Eosinophil.

SIZE: 12-17 μm
NUCLEUS: 2-3 lobes connected by thin
   filaments without visible chromatin.
Nucleoli: Not visible
Chromatin: Coarse clumped
CYTOPLASM: Pink; may have irregular
   borders
Granules:
   Primary: Rare
   Secondary: Abundant red to orange;
      round
N/C RATIO: Cytoplasm predominates
REFERENCE INTERVAL:
Bone Marrow: 0%-3%
Peripheral Blood: 0%-5%
Refer to Table 1-1 for more examples.

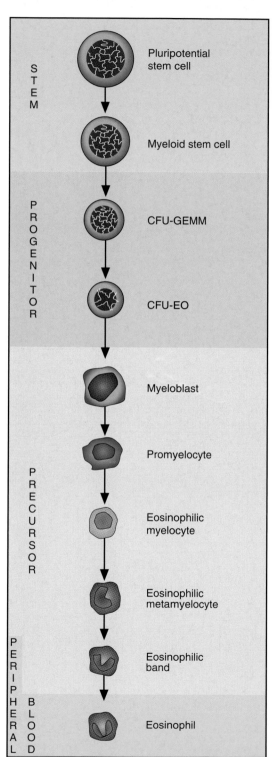

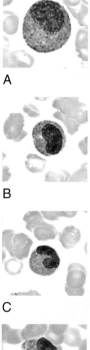

Figure 7-9 Eosinophilic sequence with **(A)** eosinophilic myelocyte, **(B)** eosinophilic metamyelocyte, **(C)** eosinophilic band, and **(D)** eosinophil.

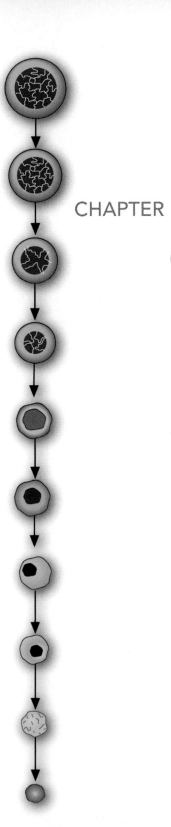

CHAPTER

8

Basophil Maturation

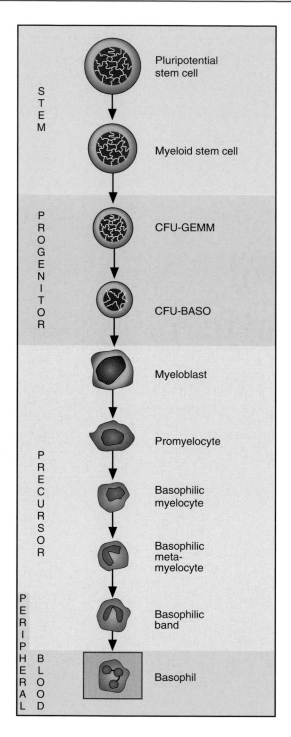

Figure 8-1 Basophilic sequence—Basophil. Stages of basophil maturation are not seen under normal conditions.

BASOPHIL

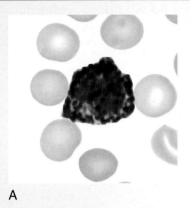

A

Figure 8-2A Basophil.

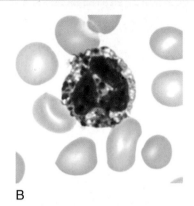

B

Figure 8-2B Basophil.

SIZE: 10-14 μm
NUCLEUS: Usually 2 lobes connected by thin
    filaments without visible chromatin
Nucleoli: Not visible
Chromatin: Coarse clumped
CYTOPLASM: Lavender to colorless
Granules:
    Primary: Rare
    Secondary: Variable in number with
        uneven distribution, may obscure
        nucleus **(A)**; deep purple to black;
        irregularly shaped. Granules are water
        soluble and may be washed out during
        staining; thus they appear as empty
        areas in the cytoplasm **(B)**.
N/C RATIO: Cytoplasm predominates.
REFERENCE INTERVAL:
Bone Marrow: <1%
Peripheral Blood: 0%-1%
Refer to Table 1-1 for more examples.

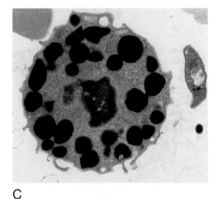

C

Figure 8-2C Electron micrograph of basophil
(×28,750).

All photomicrographs are ×1000 with Wright–Giemsa stain unless stated otherwise.

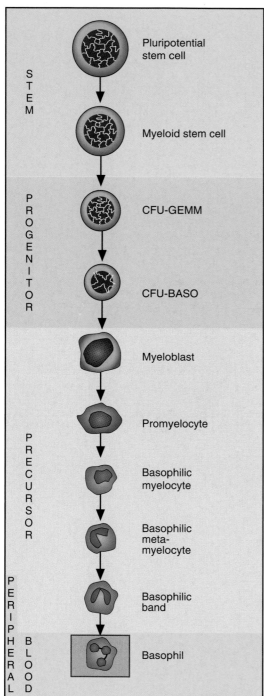

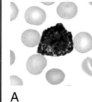

A

Figure 8-3 Maturation parallels that of the neutrophil; however, immature stages are not normally seen in normal peripheral blood. **(A)** Basophil.

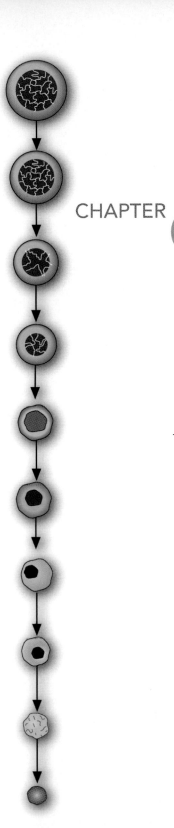

9

Lymphoid Maturation

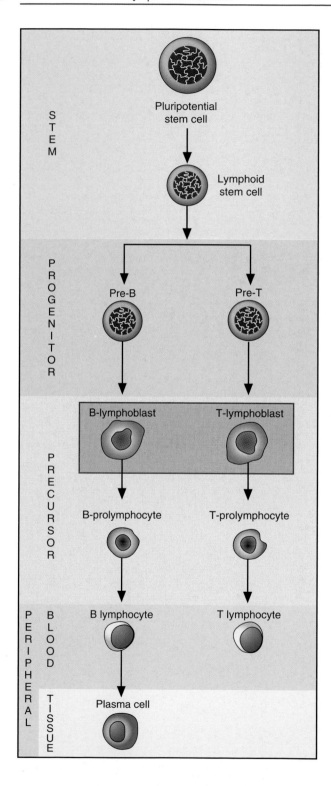

Figure 9-1 Lymphoid sequence—B lymphoblast and T lymphoblast.

LYMPHOBLAST

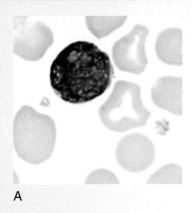

A

Figure 9-2A Lymphoblast.

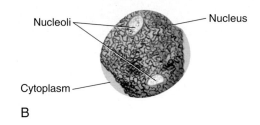

B

Figure 9-2B Schematic of lymphoblast.

SIZE: 10-18 μm
NUCLEUS: Round to oval
Nucleoli: One or more
Chromatin: Fine, evenly stained
CYTOPLASM: Moderate to deeply basophilic
Granules: None
N/C RATIO: 4:1
REFERENCE INTERVAL:
Bone Marrow: Not defined
Peripheral Blood: 0%

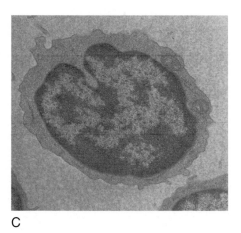

C

Figure 9-2C Electron micrograph of lymphoblast (×28,750).

All photomicrographs are ×1000 with Wright–Giemsa stain unless stated otherwise.

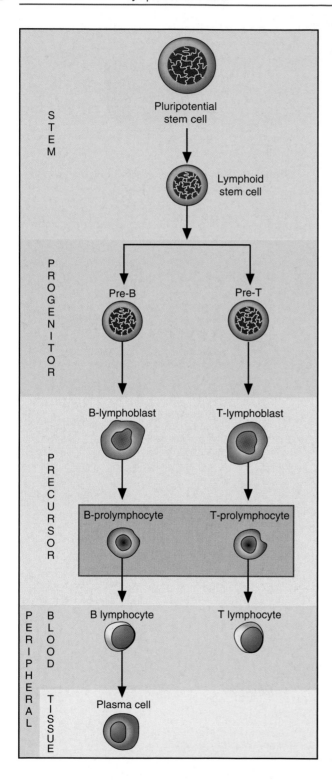

Figure 9-3 Lymphoid sequence—B and T prolymphocytes.

PROLYMPHOCYTE

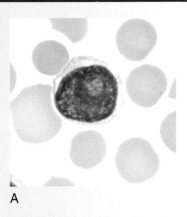

A

Figure 9-4A Prolymphocyte.

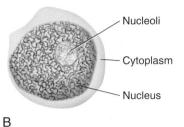

B

Figure 9-4B Schematic of prolymphocyte.

SIZE: 9-18 μm
NUCLEUS: Round or indented
Nucleoli: 0-1
Chromatin: Fine, intermediate between
   lymphoblast and mature lymphocyte
CYTOPLASM: Basophilic
Granules: None
N/C RATIO: 3-4:1
REFERENCE INTERVAL:
Bone Marrow: Not defined
Peripheral Blood: None

Prolymphocytes are difficult to distinguish morphologically in normal bone marrow.

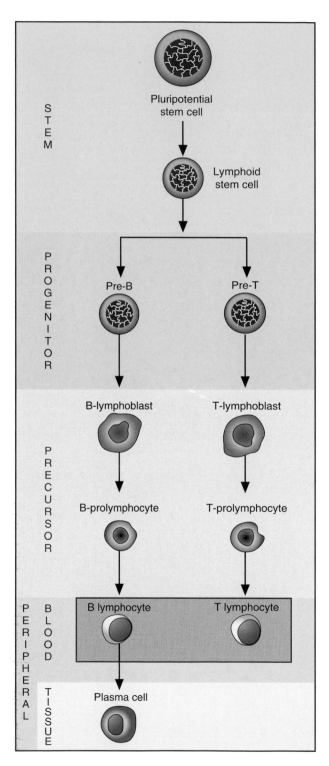

Figure 9-5 Lymphoid sequence—B and T lymphocytes. (NOTE: T lymphocytes cannot be distinguished from B lymphocytes with Wright stain.)

LYMPHOCYTE

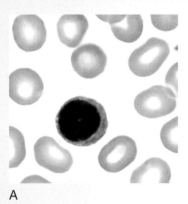

A

Figure 9-6A Small lymphocyte.

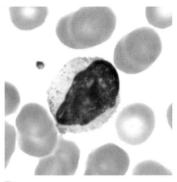

B

Figure 9-6B Large lymphocyte.

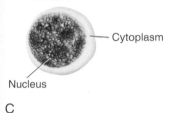

Cytoplasm

Nucleus

C

Figure 9-6C Schematic of lymphocyte.

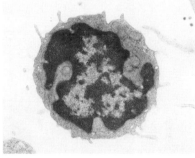

D

Figure 9-6D Electron micrograph of lympho-cyte (×30,000).

SIZE: 7-18 μm
NUCLEUS: Round to oval; may be slightly indented
Nucleoli: Occasional
Chromatin: Condensed to deeply condensed
CYTOPLASM: Scant to moderate; sky blue; vacuoles may be present
NOTE: The difference in size from small to large lymphocytes is due primarily to a larger amount of cytoplasm.
Granules: Few azurophilic (purple)
N/C RATIO: 3-5:1
REFERENCE INTERVAL:
Bone Marrow: 5%-15%
Peripheral Blood: 20%-40%
Refer to Table 1-1 for more examples.

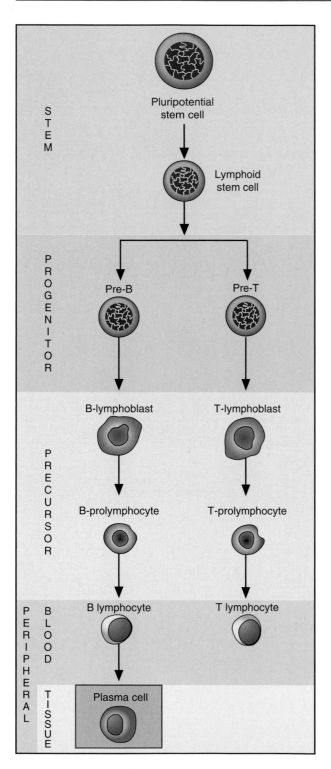

Figure 9-7 Lymphoid sequence—plasma cell.

PLASMA CELL

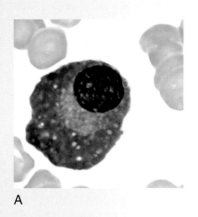

A

Figure 9-8A Plasma cell.

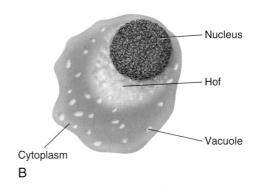

B

Figure 9-8B Schematic of plasma cell.

SIZE: 8-20 μm
NUCLEUS: Round or oval; eccentric
Nucleoli: None
Chromatin: Coarse
CYTOPLASM: Deeply basophilic, often with perinuclear clear zone (hof)
Granules: None
Vacuoles: None to several
N/C RATIO: 2-1:1
REFERENCE INTERVAL:
Bone Marrow: 0%-1%
Peripheral Blood: 0%

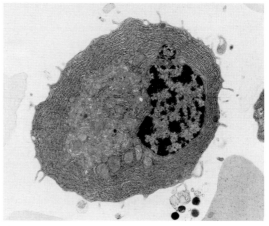

C

Figure 9-8C Electron micrograph of plasma cell (×17,500).

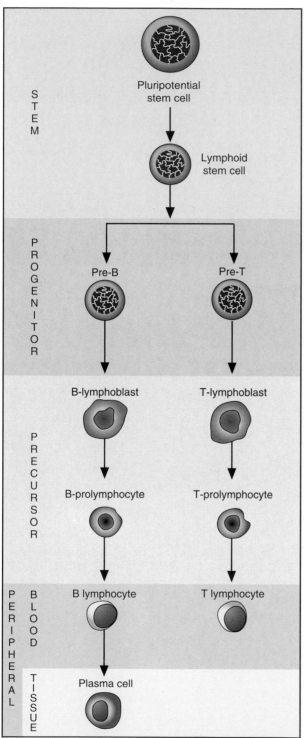

Figure 9-9 Lymphoid sequence with (A) lymphoblast, (B) prolymphocyte, (C) lymphocyte, and (D) plasma cell.

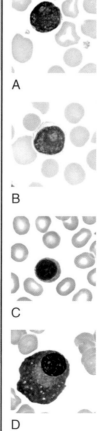

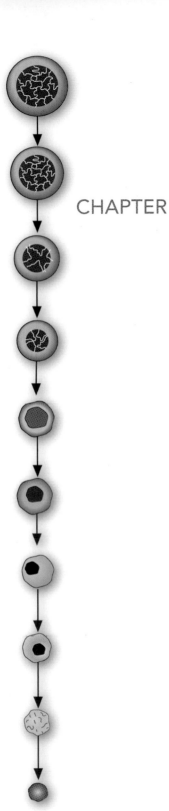

10

Variations in Size and Hemoglobin Content of Erythrocytes

VARIATIONS IN SIZE

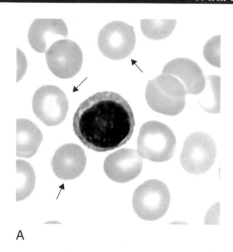

A

Figure 10-1A Microcytes. (MCV < 80 fL)

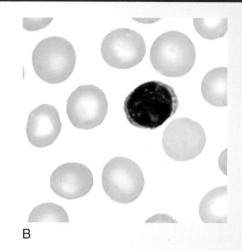

B

Figure 10-1B Normocytes. (MCV 80–100 fL)

Associated with: Iron deficiency anemia, sideroblastic anemia, thalassemia minor, chronic disease (occasionally), lead poisoning, hemoglobinopathies (some)

Normal erythrocytes are approximately the same size as the nucleus of a small lymphocyte.

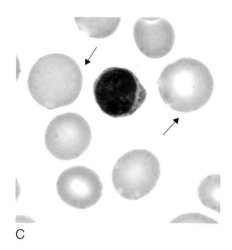

C

Figure 10-1C Macrocytes. (MCV > 100 fL)

Associated with: Liver disease, vitamin B$_{12}$ deficiency, folate deficiency, neonates

DIMORPHIC POPULATION OF ERYTHROCYTES

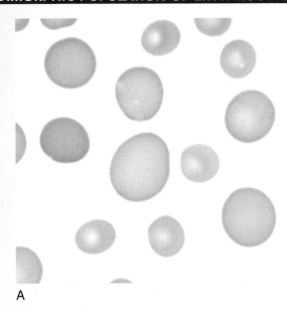

A

Figure 10-2A Dimorphic population of erythrocytes. (RDW > 14.5%)

Associated with: Transfusion, myelodysplastic syndromes, vitamin B_{12}, folate, or iron deficiencies—early in treatment process

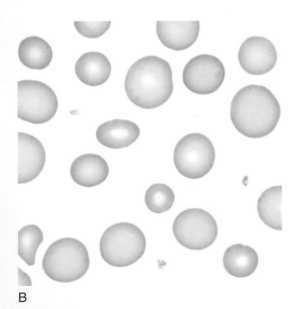

B

Figure 10-2B Dimorphic population of erythrocytes. (RDW > 14.5%)

HEMOGLOBIN CONTENT OF ERYTHROCYTES

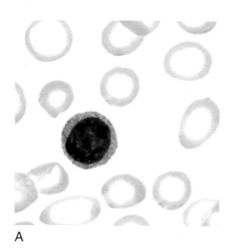

A

Figure 10-3A Hypochromia. (MCHC < 32 g/dL or 32%)

Associated with: Iron deficiency anemia, thalassemias, sideroblastic anemia, lead poisoning, some cases of chronic disease

NOTE: The central pallor zone of the erythrocyte must be greater than one third of the diameter of the cell before it is classified as hypochromic. The cells in this figure are also microcytic.

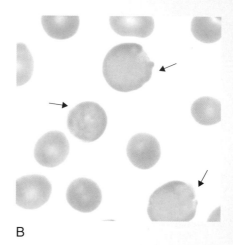

B

Figure 10-3B Polychromasia.

Associated with: Acute and chronic hemorrhage, hemolysis, effective treatment for anemia, neonates

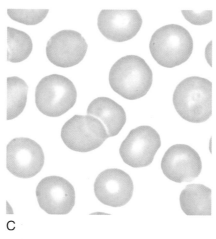

C

Figure 10-3C Normochromic erythrocytes. (MCHC 32–36 g/dL or 32%–36%)

For comparison with hypochromic and polychromatic erythrocytes

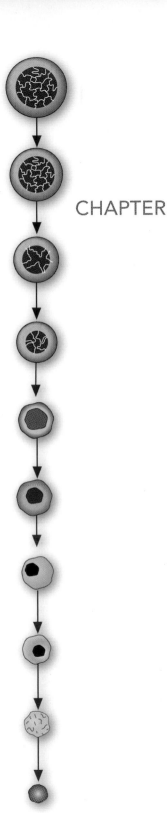

CHAPTER

11

Variations in Shape and Color of Erythrocytes

ACANTHOCYTE
Spur Cell

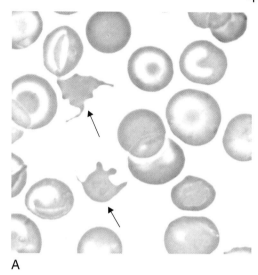

A

Figure 11-1A Acanthocyte.

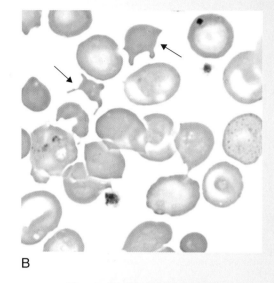

B

Figure 11-1B Acanthocyte.

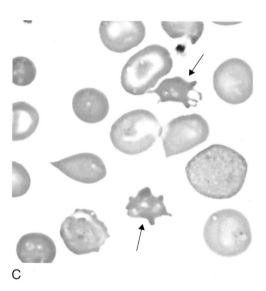

C

Figure 11-1C Acanthocyte.

Description: Erythrocyte with irregularly spaced projections that vary in width, length, and number; usually dense

Associated with: Abetalipoproteinemia, severe liver disease, splenectomy, malabsorption, hypothyroidism, vitamin E deficiency

BURR CELL
Echinocyte, Crenated Cell

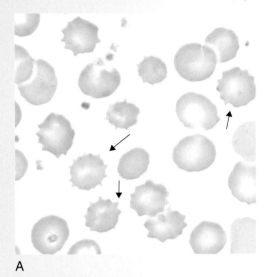

A

Figure 11-2A Burr cells.

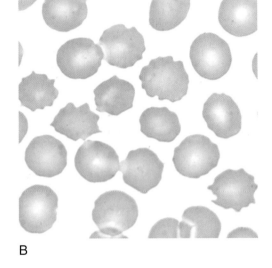

B

Figure 11-2B Burr cells.

Description: Burrlike erythrocyte with short,
  evenly spaced projections
Associated with: Uremia, pyruvate kinase
  deficiency, microangiopathic hemolytic
  anemia, neonates (especially premature),
  artifact

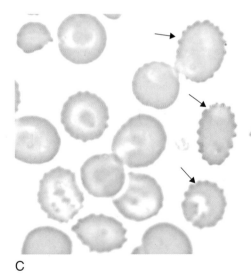

C

Figure 11-2C Burr cells.

SPHEROCYTE

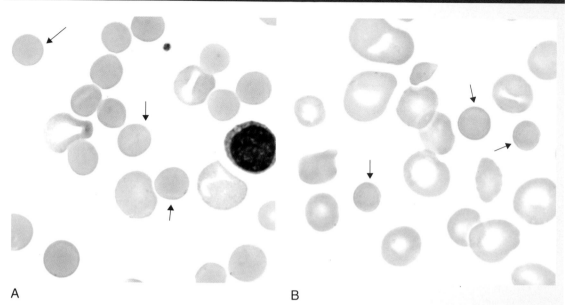

A

Figure 11-3A Spherocytes.

B

Figure 11-3B Spherocytes.

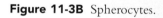

COLOR: Dark red
SHAPE: Round; no central pallor zone
Associated with: Hereditary spherocytosis, some hemolytic anemias, transfused cells, severe burns

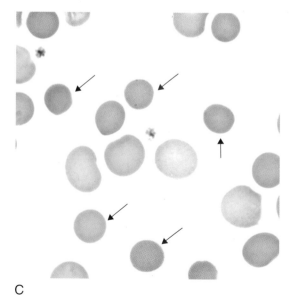

C

Figure 11-3C Spherocytes.

TARGET CELL
Codocyte

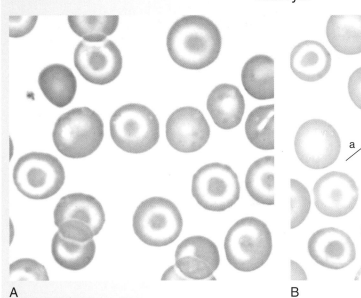

A

Figure 11-4A Target cells.

Figure 11-4B Target cells.

B

COLOR: Red to salmon

SHAPE: Bull's eye; central concentration of hemoglobin surrounded by colorless area with peripheral ring of hemoglobin resembling bull's eye; may be bell *(a)* or cup *(b)* shaped.

Associated with: Hemoglobinopathies, thalassemia, iron deficiency anemia, splenectomy, obstructive liver disease

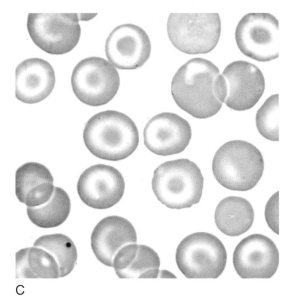

C

Figure 11-4C Target cells.

SICKLE CELL
Drepanocyte

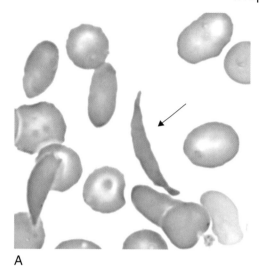

A

Figure 11-5A Sickle cell.

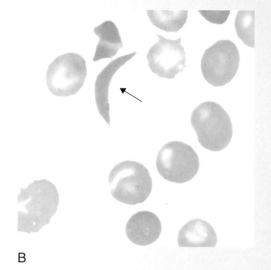

B

Figure 11-5B Sickle cell.

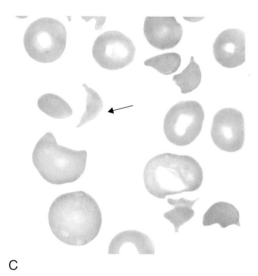

C

Figure 11-5C Schistocyte (see Figure 11–11) resembling sickle cell.

COLOR: Dark red to salmon
SHAPE: Elongated cell with point on each end; may be curved or S-shaped
COMPOSITION: Hemoglobin S
Associated with: Homozygous hemoglobin S disease

HEMOGLOBIN C CRYSTALS

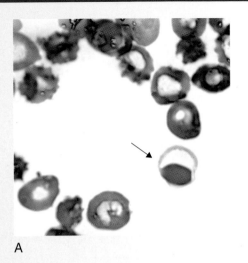

A

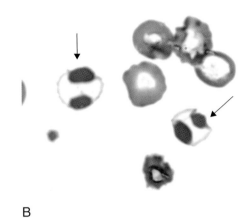

B

Figure 11-6A Induced hemoglobin C crystals (crystals induced with 3% NaCl). Note the RBC membrane around the crystals.

Figure 11-6B Induced hemoglobin C crystal (crystals induced with 3% NaCl).

COLOR: Dark red
SHAPE: Hexagonal
NUMBER PER CELL: 1 (if not induced)
COMPOSITION: Hemoglobin C
Associated with: Homozygous hemoglobin C disease

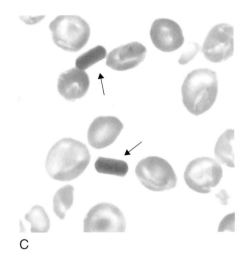

C

Figure 11-6C Hemoglobin C crystal (not induced on peripheral blood smear).

HEMOGLOBIN SC CRYSTALS

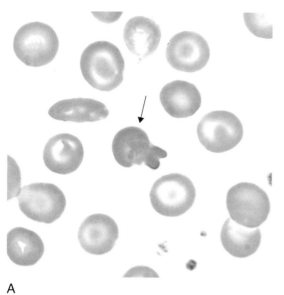

A

Figure 11-7A Hemoglobin SC crystal.

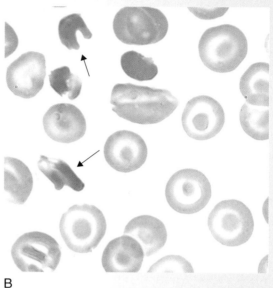

B

Figure 11-7B Hemoglobin SC crystal; note mitten shape.

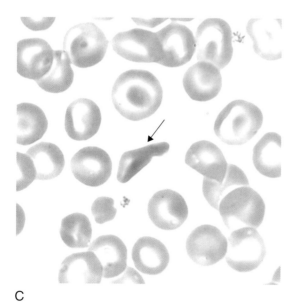

C

Figure 11-7C Hemoglobin SC crystal.

COLOR: Dark red
SHAPE: 1-2 fingerlike projections; may look like a mitten
NUMBER PER CELL: 1-2
COMPOSITION: Hemoglobin SC
Associated with: Hemoglobin SC disease

STOMATOCYTE

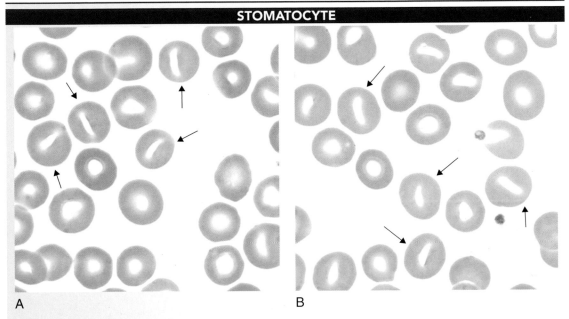

A

Figure 11-8A Stomatocytes.

B

Figure 11-8B Stomatocytes.

Description: Erythrocyte with slitlike area of central pallor (similar to a mouth or stoma)
Associated with: Hereditary stomatocytosis, alcoholism, liver disease, Rh null phenotype, artifact

ELLIPTOCYTE/OVALOCYTE

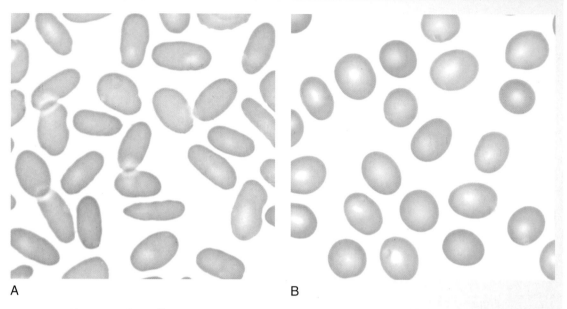

A

B

Figure 11-9A Elliptocytes.   **Figure 11-9B** Ovalocytes.

Description: Elliptocyte—cigar-shaped erythrocyte
              Ovalocyte—egg-shaped erythrocyte

Associated with: Hereditary elliptocytosis or ovalocytosis, thalassemia major, iron deficiency anemia, megaloblastic anemias (macro ovalocytes), myelophthisic anemias

TEAR DROP CELL
Dacryocyte

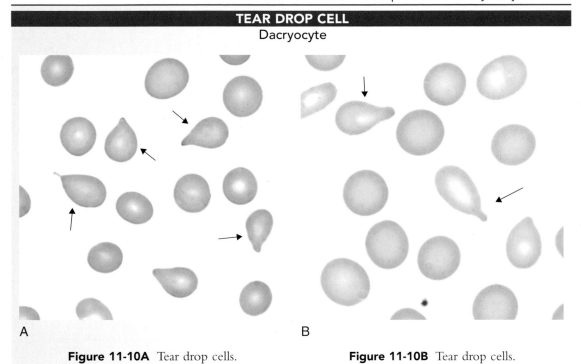

A

B

Figure 11-10A Tear drop cells.   **Figure 11-10B** Tear drop cells.

Description: Erythrocyte shaped like a tear drop or pear; may have one blunt projection
Associated with: Myelofibrosis with myeloid metaplasia, thalassemias, myelophthisic anemias, other causes of extramedullary hematopoiesis

SCHISTOCYTE
Schizocyte

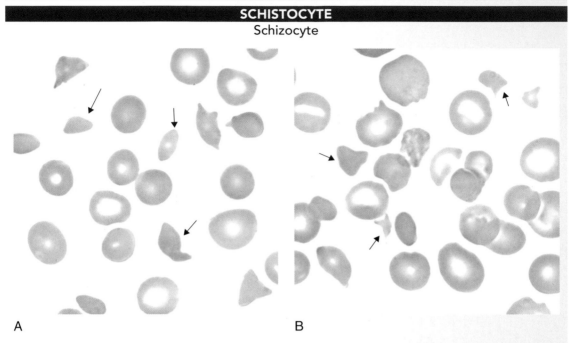

A

B

Figure 11-11A Schistocytes.   **Figure 11-11B** Schistocytes.

COLOR: Red to salmon
SHAPE: Fragmented erythrocytes; many sizes and shapes are present on a smear; often display pointed extremities
Associated with: Microangiopathic hemolytic anemia (hemolytic uremic syndrome, thrombotic thrombocytopenic purpura, disseminated intravascular coagulation), severe burns, renal graft rejection

ROULEAUX VERSUS AUTOAGGLUTINATION

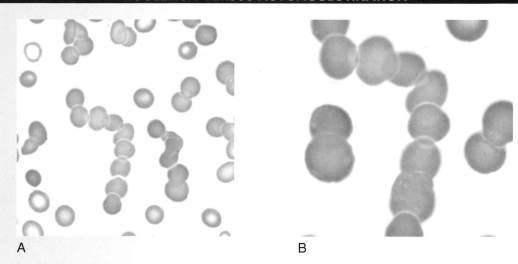

A

Figure 11-12A Rouleaux (×500).

B

Figure 11-12B Rouleaux (×1000).

ROULEAUX

Description: Erythrocytes arranged in rows like stacks of coins; increased proteins in patients with rouleaux may make the background of the slide appear blue
Associated with: Increased concentrations of globulins and/or paraproteins

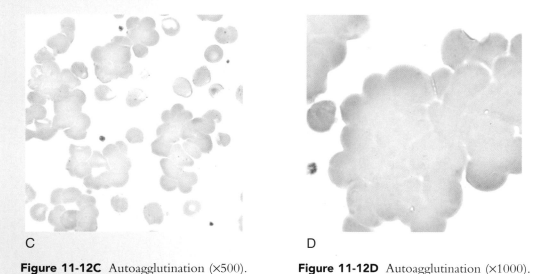

C

Figure 11-12C Autoagglutination (×500).

D

Figure 11-12D Autoagglutination (×1000).

AUTOAGGLUTINATION

Description: Clumping of erythrocytes; outlines of individual cells may not be evident
Associated with: Antigen/antibody reactions

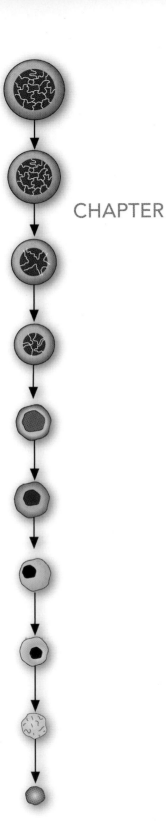

CHAPTER

12

Inclusions in Erythrocytes

TABLE 12-1 Staining Qualities of Erythrocyte Inclusion Bodies

Inclusion	Composition	Wright-Giemsa Stain	New Methylene Blue (or other Supravital Stain)	Prussian Blue (Iron)
Howell-Jolly body	DNA	+	+	0
Basophilic stippling	RNA	+	+	0
Pappenheimer body	Iron	+	+	+
Cabot ring	Remnant of mitotic spindle	+	+	0
Reticulocyte	Precipitated RNA	0	+	0
Heinz body	Unstable hemoglobin	0	+	0

+, Positive; 0, negative.

HOWELL-JOLLY BODIES

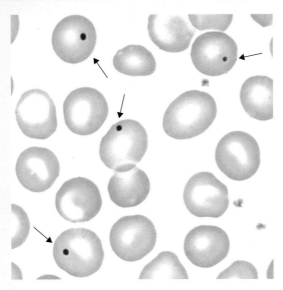

Figure 12-1 Howell-Jolly bodies.

COLOR: Dark blue to purple
SHAPE: Round to oval
SIZE: 1 μm
NUMBER PER CELL: Usually 1; may be multiple
COMPOSITION: DNA
Associated with: Splenectomy, hyposplenism, megaloblastic anemia, hemolytic anemia

BASOPHILIC STIPPLING

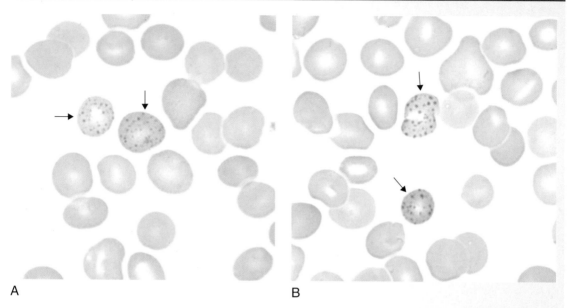

A

Figure 12-2A Basophilic stippling.

B

Figure 12-2B Basophilic stippling.

COLOR: Dark blue to purple
SHAPE: Fine or coarse granules
NUMBER PER CELL: Numerous with fairly even distribution
COMPOSITION: RNA
Associated with: Lead intoxication, thalassemia, abnormal heme synthesis

PAPPENHEIMER BODIES
Siderotic Granules

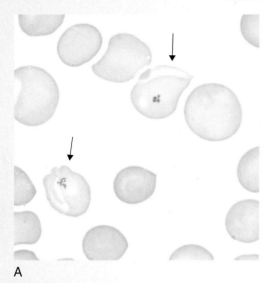

A

Figure 12-3A Pappenheimer bodies.

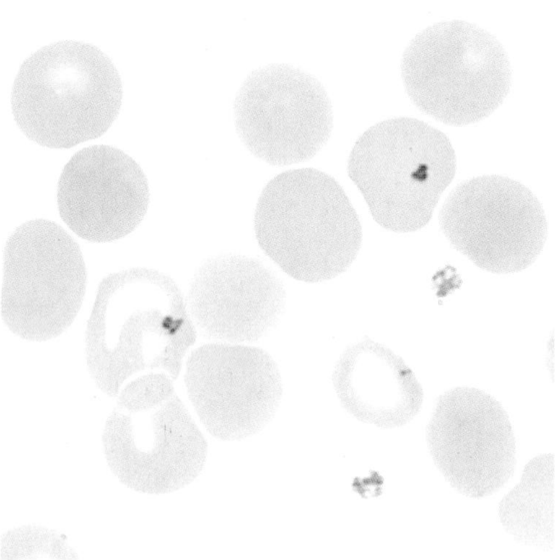

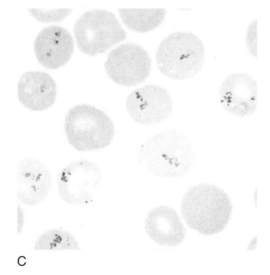

B

Figure 12-3B Pappenheimer bodies.

COLOR: Light blue
SHAPE: Fine irregular granules in clusters
NUMBER PER CELL: Usually one cluster; may be multiples; often at periphery of cell
COMPOSITION: Iron
Associated with: Splenectomy, hemolytic anemia, sideroblastic anemia, megaloblastic anemia, hemoglobinopathies

C

Figure 12-3C Siderotic granules—iron stain.

CABOT RINGS

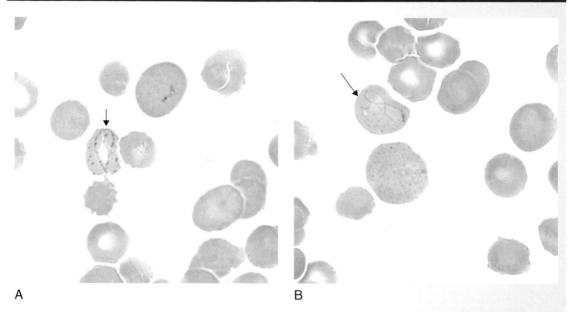

A

Figure 12-4A Cabot ring.

B

Figure 12-4B Cabot ring—figure eight.

COLOR: Dark blue to purple
SHAPE: Loop, ring, or figure eight; may look like beads on a string
NUMBER PER CELL: 1-2
COMPOSITION: Thought to be remnants of mitotic spindle
Associated with: Myelodysplastic syndrome, megaloblastic anemia

COMPARISON OF RETICULOCYTES AND HEINZ BODIES
Stained with New Methylene Blue

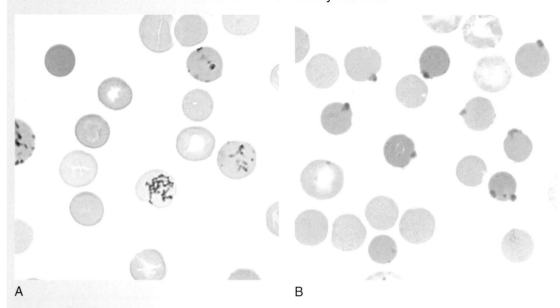

A

B

Figure 12-5A Reticulocytes.

Figure 12-5B Heinz bodies.

CELL: Anuclear immature erythrocyte
COMPOSITION: Precipitated RNA
NUMBER: ≥2 per cell
COLOR: Dark blue
Associated with: Erythrocyte maturation

CELL: Mature erythrocyte
COMPOSITION: Precipitated hemoglobin
NUMBER: Single or multiple, generally membrane bound
COLOR: Dark blue to purple
Associated with: Unstable hemoglobin, some hemoglobinopathies, some erythrocyte enzyme deficiencies (e.g., G-6-PD)
NOTE: To stimulate the formation of Heinz bodies in susceptible cells, blood may be incubated with acetylphenylhydrazine.

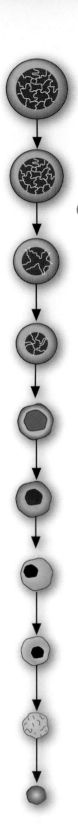

13

Diseases Affecting Erythrocytes

IRON DEFICIENCY ANEMIA

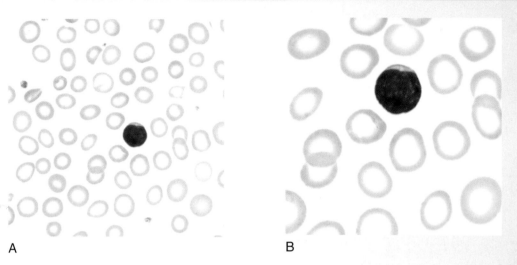

A

Figure 13-1A Iron deficiency anemia (peripheral blood [PB] ×500).

Figure 13-1B Iron deficiency anemia (PB ×1000).

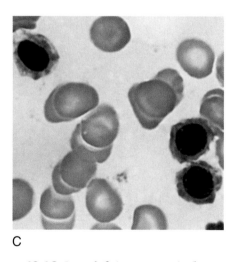

C

Figure 13-1C Iron deficiency anemia (bone marrow [BM] ×1000) (showing shaggy cytoplasm).

Peripheral Blood: Erythrocytes are hypochromic and microcytic; large variation in size; possible thrombocytosis

Bone Marrow: Erythrocyte precursors are smaller and more numerous than normal and have shaggy cytoplasm. There is nuclear cytoplasmic asynchrony, with cytoplasmic maturation lagging behind that of the nucleus.

Although characteristic findings for disease states are listed, not all may be present in one patient. The most common ones are depicted.

α AND β THALASSEMIA MINOR

$$-/\alpha\alpha-\quad -\alpha/-\alpha\quad -/\alpha\alpha$$
$$\beta/\beta^0\quad \beta/\beta^+\quad \beta/(\delta\beta)^0\quad \beta/(\delta\beta)\text{Lepore}$$

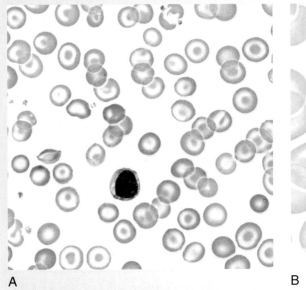

A

Figure 13-2A Thalassemia minor (PB ×500).

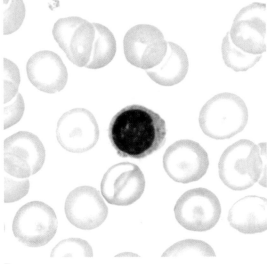

B

Figure 13-2B Thalassemia minor (PB ×1000).

Peripheral Blood: Microcytosis, slight hypochromia, target cells, basophilic stippling

β–THALASSEMIA MAJOR

β⁰β⁰   β⁺β⁺   β⁰β⁺   (δβ)Lepore/(δβ)Lepore

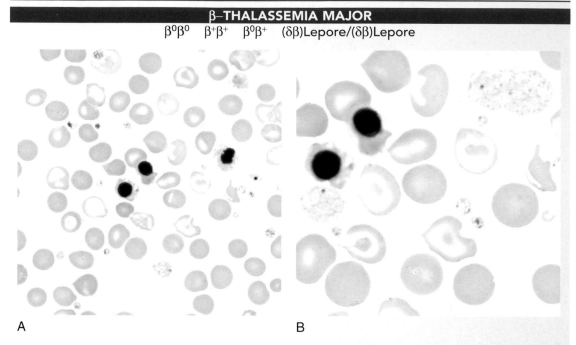

A

B

Figure 13-3A β-Thalassemia major (PB ×500).   **Figure 13-3B** β-Thalassemia major (PB ×1000).

Peripheral Blood: Numerous nucleated erythrocytes, microcytes, hypochromia, target cells, basophilic stippling, many tear drop cells, many schistocytes, polychromasia

BART'S HEMOGLOBIN
(4 α–Chain Deletion)

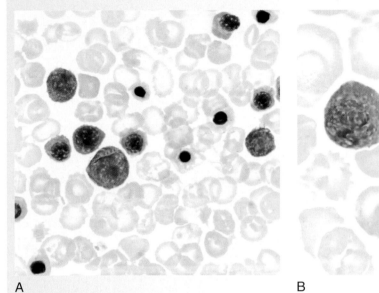 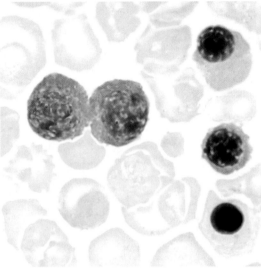

A

B

Figure 13-4A Bart's hemoglobin (PB ×500).   **Figure 13-4B** Bart's hemoglobin (PB ×1000).

Peripheral Blood: Marked variation in size, hypochromia, numerous nucleated erythrocytes, variable polychromasia, macrocytes

MACROCYTIC ANEMIA
Nonmegaloblastic

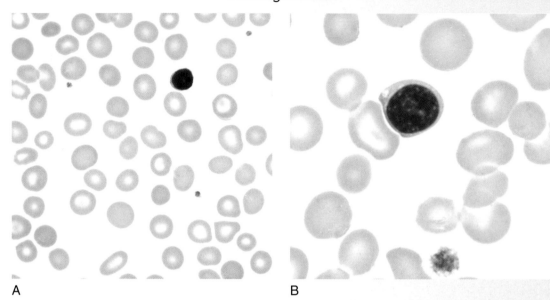

A

B

Figure 13-5A Macrocytic (nonmegaloblastic) (PB ×500).

Figure 13-5B Macrocytic (nonmegaloblastic) (PB ×1000).

Peripheral Blood: Round macrocytes, leukocyte and platelet counts usually normal
Bone Marrow: No megaloblastic changes

MEGALOBLASTIC ANEMIA

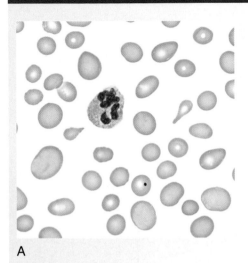

A

Figure 13-6A Megaloblastic anemia (PB ×500).

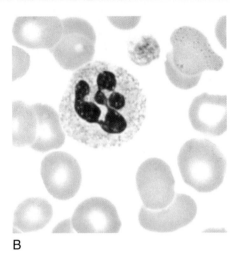

B

Figure 13-6B Megaloblastic anemia (PB ×1000).

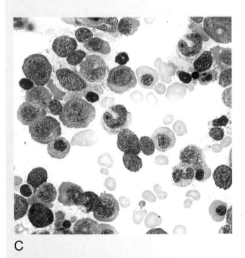

C

Figure 13-6C Megaloblastic anemia (BM original ×500).

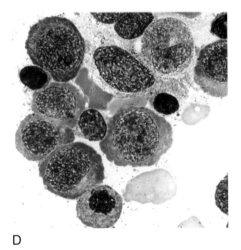

D

Figure 13-6D Megaloblastic anemia (BM original ×1000).

Peripheral Blood: Pancytopenia, oval macrocytes, Howell-Jolly bodies, nucleated erythrocytes, basophilic stippling, hypersegmentation of neutrophils, giant platelets, target cells, schistocytes, spherocytes, tear drop cells

NOTE: Triad of abnormalities: Oval macrocytes, hypersegmented neutrophils, and Howell-Jolly bodies.

Bone Marrow: Hypercellular, asynchrony (trilineage), giant bands, giant metamyelocytes, hypersegmented megakaryocytes

APLASTIC ANEMIA

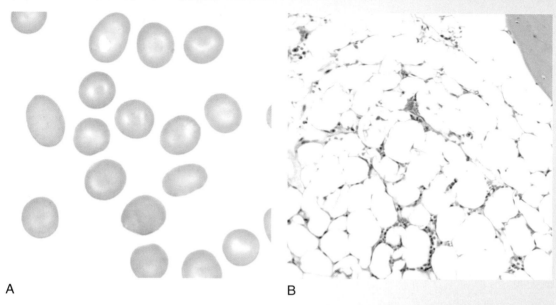

A

Figure 13-7A Aplastic anemia (PB ×1000).

B

Figure 13-7B Aplastic anemia (BM biopsy ×1000).

Peripheral Blood: Pancytopenia, normocytic, normochromic (occasional macrocytes)
Bone Marrow: Hypocellular; lymphocytes may predominate

IMMUNE HEMOLYTIC ANEMIA

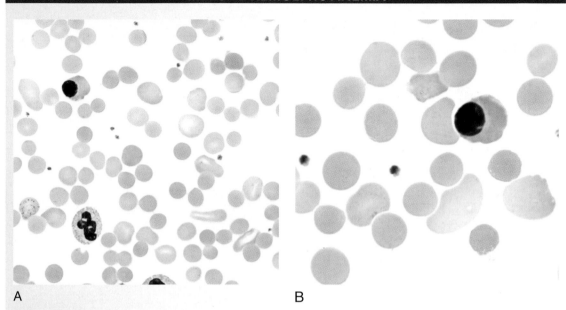

A

B

Figure 13-8A Immune hemolytic anemia (PB ×500).

Figure 13-8B Immune hemolytic anemia (PB ×1000).

Peripheral Blood: Spherocytes, schistocytes, polychromasia, nucleated erythrocytes
NOTE: Erythrocyte morphology varies with cause and severity of disease.

HEMOLYTIC DISEASE OF THE NEWBORN

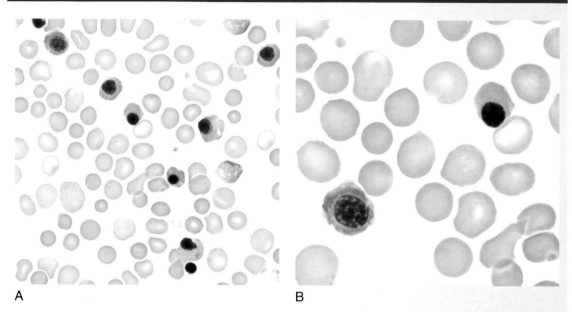

A

B

Figure 13-9A Hemolytic disease of the newborn (PB ×500).

Figure 13-9B Hemolytic disease of the newborn (PB ×1000).

Peripheral Blood: Increased number of nucleated erythrocytes, macrocytic/normochromic, polychromasia, spherocytes

NOTE: Normal newborns have some nucleated erythrocytes (see Chapter 24).

HEREDITARY SPHEROCYTOSIS

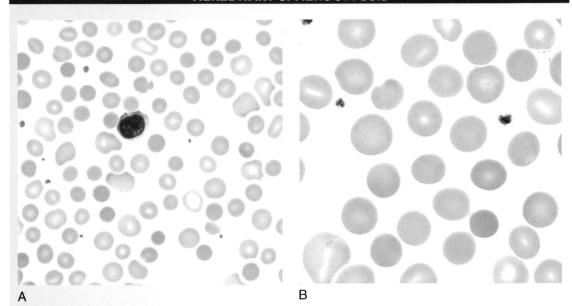

A

B

Figure 13-10A Hereditary spherocytosis (PB ×500).

Figure 13-10B Hereditary spherocytosis (PB ×1000).

Peripheral Blood: Spherocytes (variable in number), polychromasia; nucleated erythrocytes possible

HEREDITARY ELLIPTOCYTOSIS

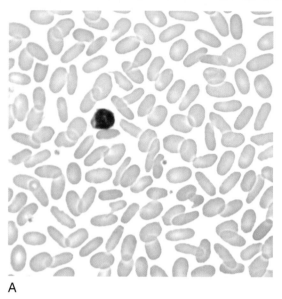

A

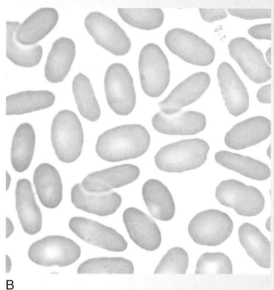

B

Figure 13-11A Hereditary elliptocytosis (PB ×500).

Figure 13-11B Hereditary elliptocytosis (PB ×1000).

Peripheral Blood: >25% elliptocytes, usually >60% elliptocytes; indices are normocytic, normochromic

NOTE: Hemolytic variant of hereditary elliptocytosis: Microelliptocytes, schistoctyes, spherocytes.

MICROANGIOPATHIC HEMOLYTIC ANEMIA (MAHA)

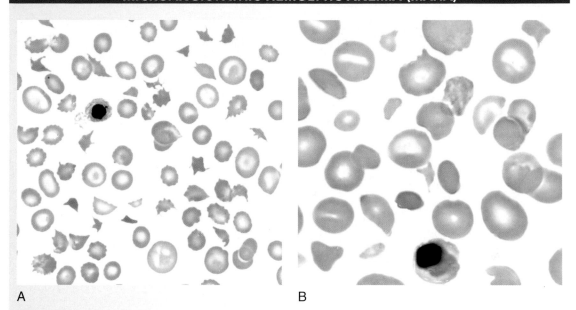

A

B

Figure 13-12A Microangiopathic hemolytic anemia (PB ×500).

Figure 13-12B Microangiopathic hemolytic anemia (PB ×1000).

Peripheral Blood: Schistocytes, spherocytes, polychromasia, nucleated erythrocytes, decreased platelet count

NOTE: The degree of morphological change correlates directly with severity of the disease.

HEMOGLOBIN CC DISEASE

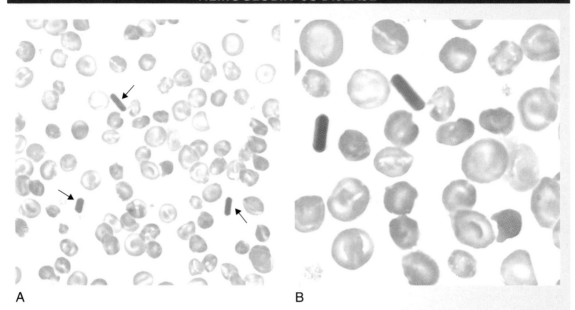

A

B

Figure 13-13A Hemoglobin CC (PB ×500).

Figure 13-13B Hemoglobin CC (PB ×1000).

Peripheral Blood: Target cells, spherocytes, microcytes, polychromasia, intracellular and/or rod-shaped crystals possible

HEMOGLOBIN SS DISEASE

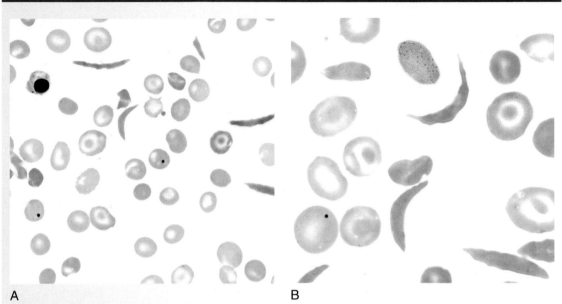

A

B

Figure 13-14A Hemoglobin SS (PB ×500).

Figure 13-14B Hemoglobin SS (PB ×1000).

Peripheral Blood: Sickle cells (in crises), target cells, nucleated erythrocytes, schistocytes, Howell-Jolly bodies, basophilic stippling, polychromasia, increased leukocyte count with neutrophilia, increased platelet count

HEMOGLOBIN SC DISEASE

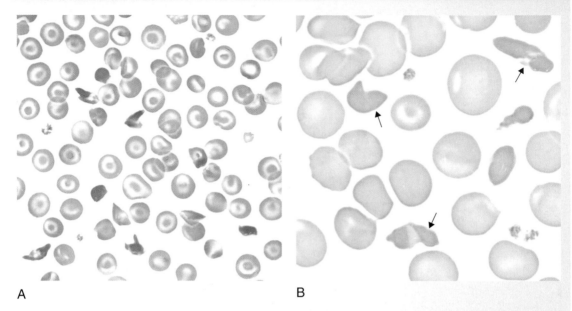

A

Figure 13-15A Hemoglobin SC (PB ×500).

B

Figure 13-15B Hemoglobin SC (PB ×1000).

PERIPHERAL BLOOD: Few sickle cells, target cells, intraerythrocytic crystals. Crystalline aggregates of hemoglobin SC may protrude from the erythrocyte membrane.

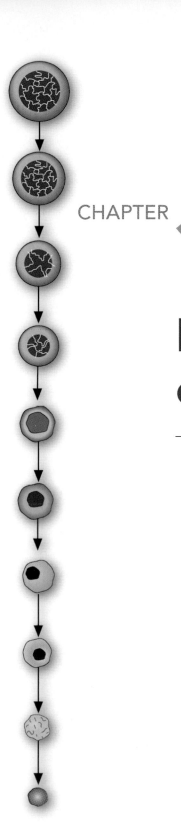

14

Nuclear Alterations of Leukocytes

HYPOSEGMENTATION

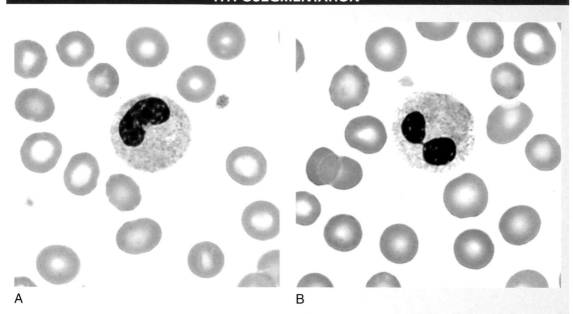

A

B

Figure 14-1A Hyposegmentation—peanut shaped (PB × 1000).

Figure 14-1B Hyposegmentation—bilobed shape (PB × 1000).

DESCRIPTION: Bilobed or peanut-shaped neutrophil nucleus with coarse chromatin
Associated with: Pelger-Huët anomaly, myeloproliferative or myelodysplastic disorders

HYPERSEGMENTATION

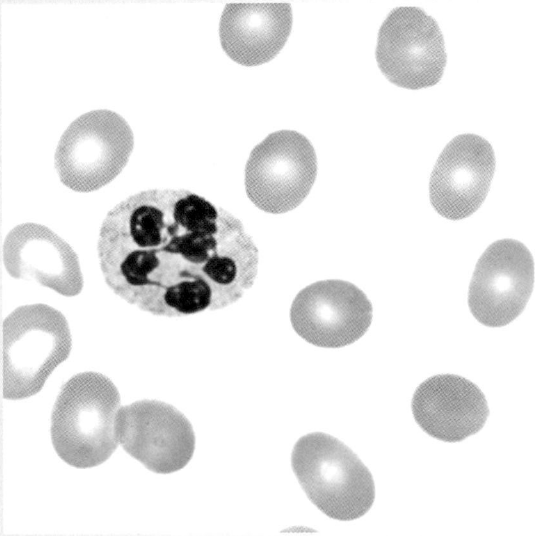

A

Figure 14-2A Hypersegmentation (PB × 1000).

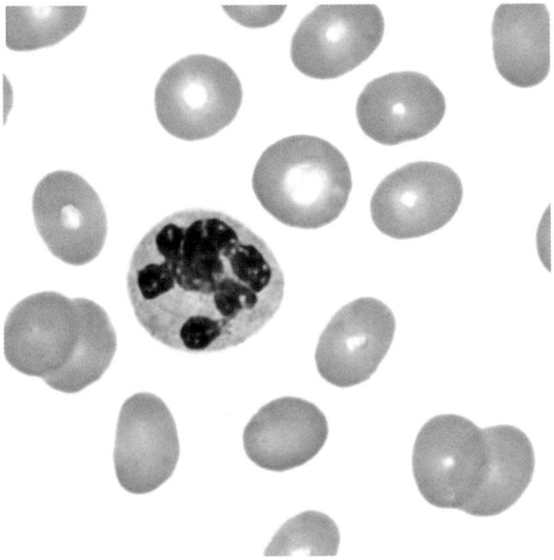

B

Figure 14-2B Hypersegmentation (PB × 1000).

DESCRIPTION: Six or more lobes in neutrophil nucleus
Associated with: Megaloblastic anemias; chronic infections; rarely inherited

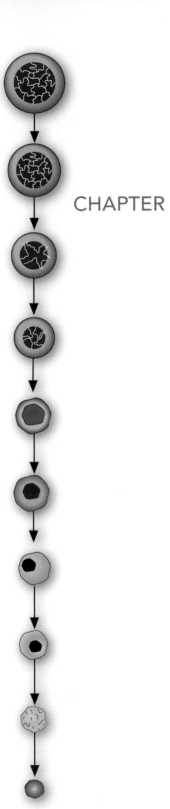

15

Cytoplasmic Alterations of Leukocytes

VACUOLIZATION

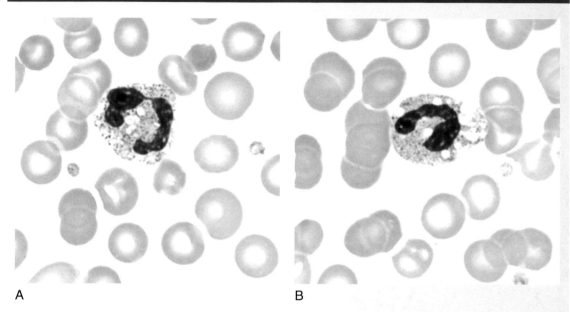

A

B

Figure 15-1A Vacuoles.

Figure 15-1B Vacuoles.

DESCRIPTION: Unstained circular area; usually within the cytoplasm
NUMBER: Few to many
Associated with: Bacterial or fungal infection, poisoning, burns, chemotherapy, artifact

All photomicrographs are ×1000 with Wright–Giemsa stain unless stated otherwise.

DÖHLE BODY

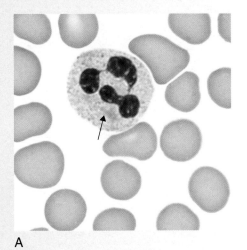

A

Figure 15-2A Döhle body.

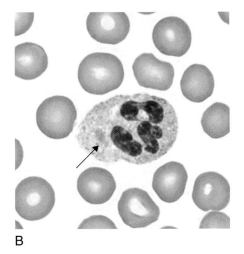

B

Figure 15-2B Döhle body.

DESCRIPTION: Gray-blue round or oval body
LOCATION: Cytoplasm, often near periphery
COMPOSITION: Ribosomal RNA
NUMBER: Single or multiple
Associated with: Bacterial infection, poisoning, burns, chemotherapy, May-Hegglin anomaly, pregnancy

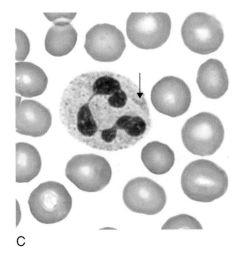

C

Figure 15-2C Döhle body.

TOXIC GRANULATION

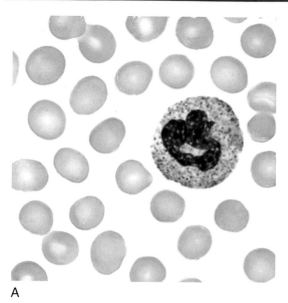

A

Figure 15-3A Toxic granulation.

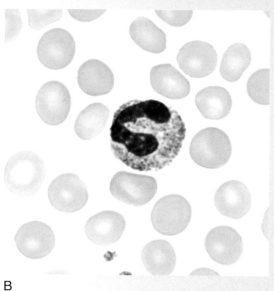

B

Figure 15-3B Toxic granulation.

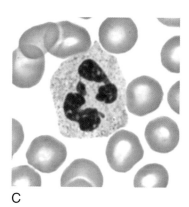

C

Figure 15-3C Normal polymorphonuclear neutrophil.

DESCRIPTION: Prominent blue-black granules
LOCATION: Cytoplasm of neutrophils, unevenly distributed
COMPOSITION: Primary granules
NUMBER: Few to many
Associated with: Bacterial infection, poisoning, burns, chemotherapy, pregnancy

DEGRANULATION/AGRANULATION

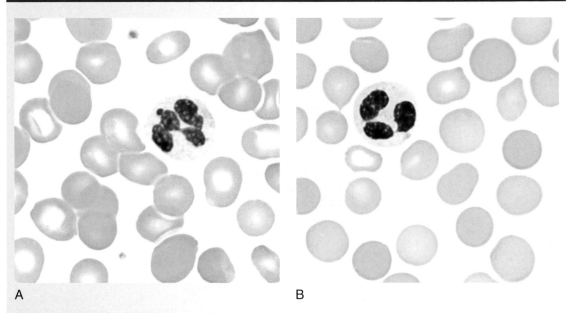

A

B

Figure 15-4A Degranulation.

Figure 15-4B Agranulation.

DESCRIPTION: Decreased number or absence of specific granules
Associated with: Infection, myelodysplastic syndrome

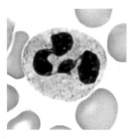

Normal neutrophil for comparison.

ERYTHROPHAGOCYTOSIS

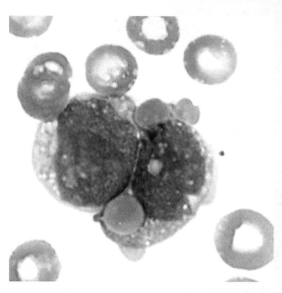

Figure 15-5 Erythrophagocytosis.

DESCRIPTION: Monocyte or macrophage that has engulfed an erythrocyte
Associated with: Familial hemophagocytic histiocytosis; idiopathic

GAUCHER DISEASE

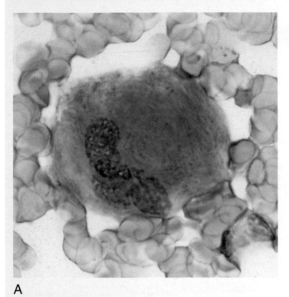

A

B

Figure 15-6A Gaucher cell.

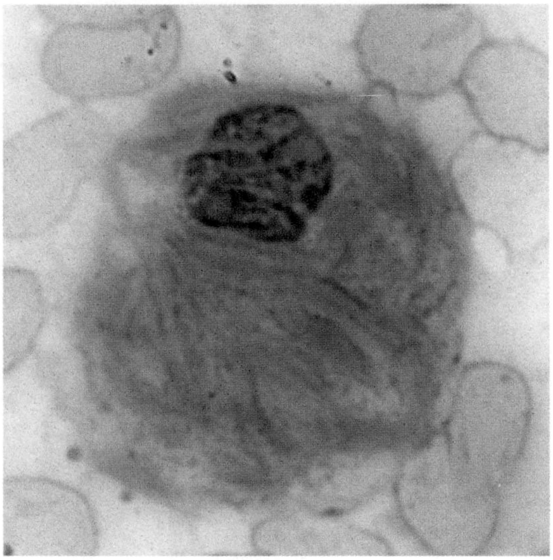

Figure 15-6B Gaucher cell.

DESCRIPTION: The Gaucher cell is a macrophage 20 to 80 μm in diameter, with one or more small, round to oval eccentric nuclei; cytoplasm has crumpled tissue paper appearance; found in bone marrow, spleen, liver, and other affected tissue

NIEMANN-PICK DISEASE

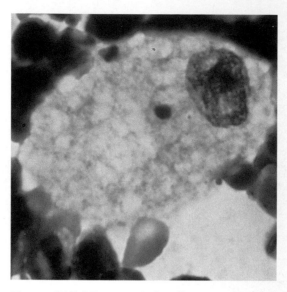

Figure 15-7 Niemann–Pick cell.

DESCRIPTION: The Niemann-Pick cell is a macrophage, 20 to 90 μm in diameter, with a small eccentric nucleus and foamy cytoplasm. It is found in bone marrow and lymphoid tissue. The peripheral blood of patients with Niemann-Pick disease may exhibit vacuolated lymphocytes.

SEA BLUE HISTIOCYTE

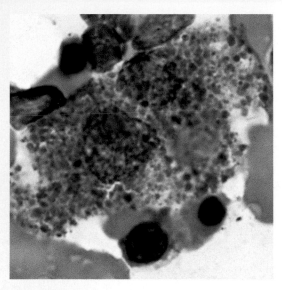

Figure 15-8 Sea blue histiocyte.

DESCRIPTION: The sea blue histiocyte is a macrophage 20 to 60 μm in diameter with an eccentric nucleus. The cytoplasm contains varying numbers of prominent blue-green granules. These cells are found in spleen, liver, and bone marrow.

Associated with: Familial sea blue histiocytosis, myeloproliferative diseases

MAY-HEGGLIN ANOMALY

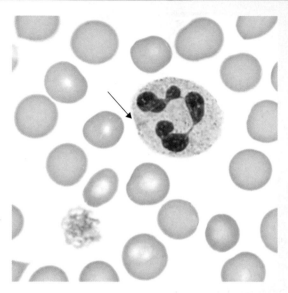

Figure 15-9 May-Hegglin anomaly.

DESCRIPTION: This anomaly is characterized by thrombocytopenia with large and/or bizarre platelets and large inclusions resembling Döhle bodies in all leukocytes with the absence of toxic granulation.

NOTE: These inclusions are sporadically visible by light microscopy but always detectable by electron microscopy.

CHÉDIAK-HIGASHI ANOMALY

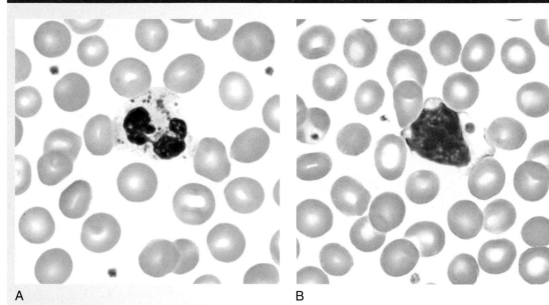

A

Figure 15-10A Chédiak–Higashi anomaly; neutrophil with granules.

B

Figure 15-10B Chédiak–Higashi anomaly; lymphocyte with granule.

DESCRIPTION: Large gray-blue granules in the cytoplasm of many monocytes and granulocytes. Lymphocytes may contain large red-purple granules.

ALDER REILLY ANOMALY

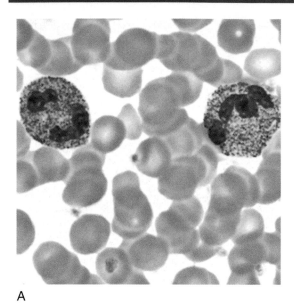

A

B

Figure 15-11A Alder Reilly anomaly. (Courtesy Dennis P. O'Malley, MD; US Labs, Irvine, Calif.)

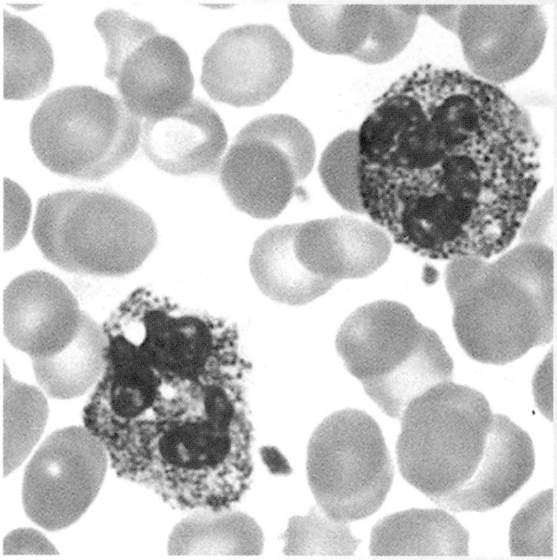

Figure 15-11B Alder Reilly anomaly. (Courtesy Dennis P. O'Malley, MD; US Labs, Irvine, Calif.)

DESCRIPTION: Deep purple to lilac granules difficult to distinguish from toxic granulation; occur in neutrophils and occasionally eosinophils and basophils.
Associated with: Hurler and Hunter syndromes

AÜER RODS

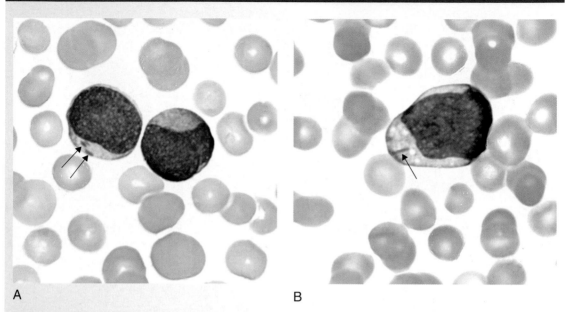

A

B

Figure 15-12A Aüer rods.   **Figure 15-12B** Aüer rod.

DESCRIPTION: Fused primary granules; usually rods; occasionally round
COLOR: Red
LOCATION: Cytoplasm
NUMBER: Single or multiple
Associated with: Acute leukemia in leukemic myeloblasts and promyelocytes—FAB[†] M1 through M6

[†]French-American-British classification of acute leukemia.

REACTIVE LYMPHOCYTES

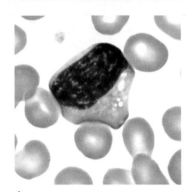

A

Figure 15-13A Reactive lymphocyte, vacuolated cytoplasm.

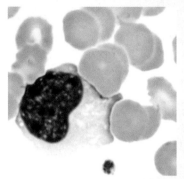

B

Figure 15-13B Reactive lymphocyte, peripheral basophilia.

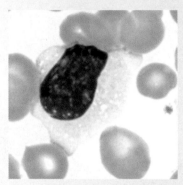

C

Figure 15-13C Reactive lymphocytes, cytoplasm indented by adjacent cells.

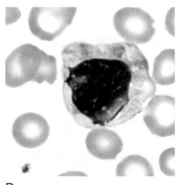

D

Figure 15-13D Reactive lymphocyte, radial basophilia.

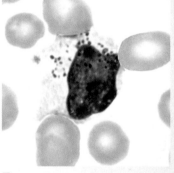

E

Figure 15-13E Reactive lymphocyte, large azurophilic granules.

SHAPE: Pleomorphic; easily indented by surrounding cells
SIZE: 10-30 μm
NUCLEUS: Irregular
  Nucleoli: Occasionally present
  Chromatin: When compared with that of a resting lymphocyte, chromatin pattern is less dense and may be fine and dispersed.
CYTOPLASM: Pale blue to deeply basophilic, may stain unevenly with peripheral or radial basophilia
  Granules: May have increased numbers of azurophilic granules
  Vacuoles: Occasionally
Associated with: Viral infections and other antigenic stimulation, including organ transplantation
NOTE: Although reactive lymphocytes display changes in both nucleus and cytoplasm, they are included in this chapter because the cytoplasmic changes are the more prominent feature.

TABLE 15-1 Monocyte versus Reactive Lymphocyte

	Monocyte	Reactive Lymphocyte
Shape	Pleomorphic; may have pseudopodia, which tend to "push away" surrounding cells	Pleomorphic, easily indented by surrounding cells
Size	12-20 µm	10-30 µm
Nucleus	Round, oval, horseshoe, or kidney shaped, may have brainlike convolutions	Irregular, elongated, stretched, occasionally round
Nucleoli	Absent	Occasionally present
Chromatin	Loosely woven, lacy	Variable; clumped to fine and dispersed
Cytoplasm	Blue-gray	Pale blue to deeply basophilic, may stain unevenly
Granules	Many fine red—may give ground glass appearance	May be a few prominent azurophilic granules
Vacuoles	Absent to numerous	Occasional

Use as many criteria as possible to identify cells. It is often difficult to differentiate cells in isolation; multiple fields should be examined for nuclear and cytoplasmic characteristics. Consider "the company they keep."

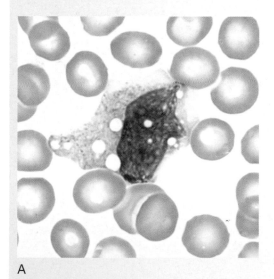

A

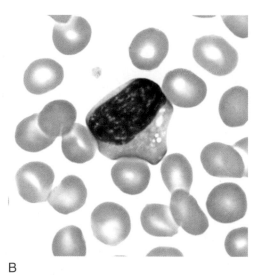

B

Figure 15-14A Monocyte. Note the blue–gray cytoplasm with fine red granules. Nucleus has brainlike convolutions. Cell "pushes away" surrounding cells. Vacuoles are present in both of these cells.

Figure 15-14B Reactive lymphocyte. Note the blue cytoplasm with darker blue periphery. Cell is indented by surrounding cells. Nucleus is elongated. Vacuoles are present in both of these cells.

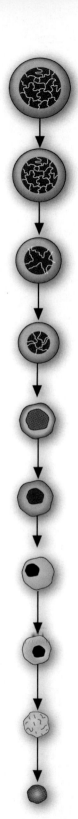

CHAPTER

16

Acute Myeloid Leukemia

Since the early 1980s, the French–American–British (FAB) classification of the acute leukemias, myeloproliferative disorders, and myelodysplastic syndromes has been widely used. The FAB system was based primarily on morphologic criteria and cytochemical reactions. However, there were flaws in this system, especially with the inability to differentiate among the lymphoid leukemias using cytochemistry.

Advances in technology have expanded the tools for diagnosis and/or prognosis and treatment, and it became clear that a new classification system was needed. In 1995 the World Health Organization (WHO) developed a classification system based on morphology; immunophenotyping; genetic features, including karyotype and molecular testing; and clinical features. Among the changes in classification is the reduction of blasts necessary for diagnosis of acute leukemia from 30% to 20%. The WHO system has been widely published, and the reader is referred to the WHO publication* or to journal articles that discuss the system.

Since this is a morphology atlas and a detailed discussion of classification systems is beyond the scope of this book, we will continue to portray the cytological characteristics with the understanding that only one criterion is being presented. Simple boxes will be incorporated where appropriate.

---

*From Jaffe ES, Harris NL, Stein H, Vardiman JW, editors: World Health Organization classification of tumors: pathology and genetics of tumors of haematopoietic and lymphoid tissues, Lyon, France, 2001, IARC Press.

BOX 16-1 Acute Myeloid Leukemias

FAB classification
- M0 through M7

WHO classification
- Acute myeloid leukemias with recurrent cytogenetic translocations
  - Acute promyelocytic leukemia (FAB M3) is included in this group, with the characteristic finding of t(15;17)(q22;q11-12) and variants, PML/RARA
- Acute myeloid leukemia with multilineage dysplasia
- Acute myeloid leukemia and myelodysplasia, therapy related
- Acute myeloid leukemia, not otherwise categorized
  - FAB M0 through M7, with the exception of FAB M3 and M4Eo, are included in this group.

FAB, French-American-British; *WHO*, World Health Organization

ACUTE MYELOID LEUKEMIA, MINIMALLY DIFFERENTIATED
FAB* M0

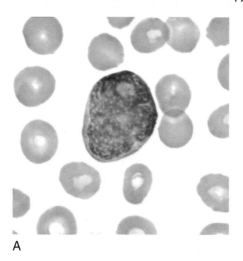

A

Figure 16-1A Peripheral blood (×1000).

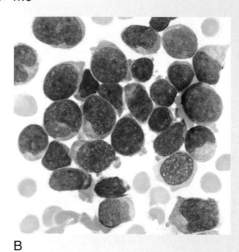

B

Figure 16-1B Bone marrow (×500).

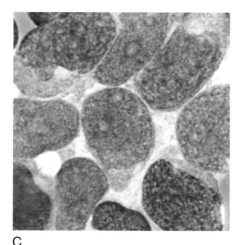

C

Figure 16-1C Bone marrow (×1000).

Peripheral Blood: Large agranular blasts, thrombocytopenia

Bone Marrow: >20% blasts all nucleated cells (ANC), >90% blasts nonerythroid cells (NEC), myeloperoxidase (MPX)-negative (see Figure 21-1A), Sudan Black B (SBB)-negative (see Figure 21-1B)

---

*French–American–British classification of acute leukemias.

ACUTE MYELOID LEUKEMIA WITHOUT DIFFERENTIATION
FAB M1

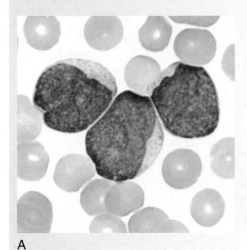

A

Figure 16-2A Peripheral blood (×1000).

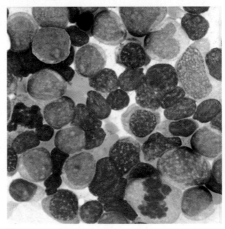

B

Figure 16-2B Bone marrow (×500).

Peripheral Blood: Blasts, thrombocytopenia
  ± Auer rods (see Figure 15-12)
Bone Marrow: >20% blasts ANC, >90%
  blasts NEC, MPX/SBB-positive in ≥3% cells
  (see Figures 21-1A and 21-1B)

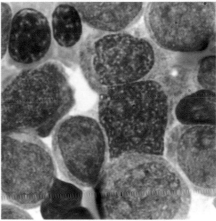

C

Figure 16-2C Bone marrow (×1000).

ACUTE MYELOID LEUKEMIA WITH DIFFERENTIATION
FAB M2

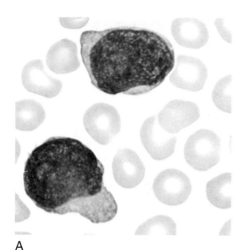

A

Figure 16-3A Peripheral blood (×1000).

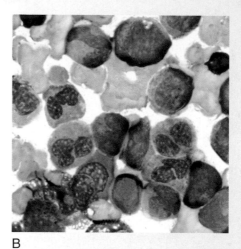

B

Figure 16-3B Bone marrow (×500).

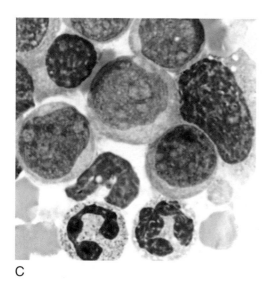

C

Figure 16-3C Bone marrow (×1000).

Peripheral Blood: Blasts with some maturation, ±Auer rods, thrombocytopenia

Bone Marrow: >20% blasts ANC, <90% blasts NEC, >10% granulocytic component, <20% monocytic component, maturation beyond promyelocyte stage in >10% of NEC, MPX/SBB-positive in ≥3% cells (see Figures 21-1A and 21-1B), ±Auer rods

ACUTE PROMYELOCYTIC LEUKEMIA
FAB M3

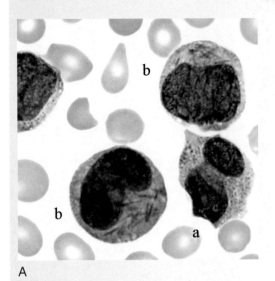

A

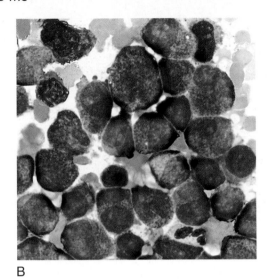

B

Figure 16-4A Peripheral blood. *a*, Hypergranular promyelocyte (×1000); *b*, Faggot cells.

Figure 16-4B Bone marrow (×500).

Peripheral Blood: Hypergranular promyelocytes, nuclei often bilobed or kidney-shaped, multiple Auer rods possible, may be in bundles (Faggot cells)

Bone Marrow: Hypergranular promyelocytes, nuclei often bilobed or kidney-shaped, multiple Auer rods; MPX/SBB—strongly positive (see Figures 21-1A and 21-1B)

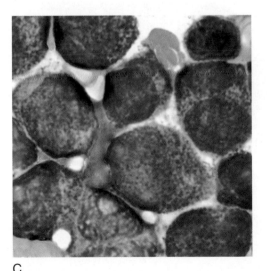

C

Figure 16-4C Bone marrow (×1000).

ACUTE PROMYELOCYTIC LEUKEMIA—MICROGRANULAR VARIANT
FAB M3m

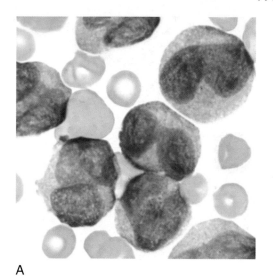

A

Figure 16-5A Peripheral blood (×1000).

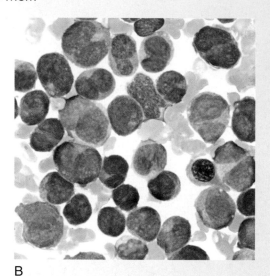

B

Figure 16-5B Bone marrow (×500).

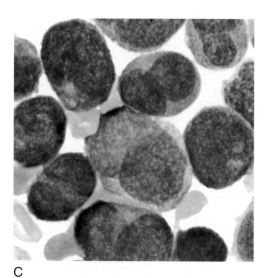

C

Figure 16-5C Bone marrow (×1000).

Peripheral Blood: Deeply notched nuclei; granules not visible by light microscopy but may be seen on electron microscopy (EM)

Bone Marrow: Agranular promyelocytes, with deeply notched nuclei, MPX/SBB—strongly positive (see Figures 21-1A and 21-1B)

ACUTE MYELOMONOCYTIC LEUKEMIA
FAB M4

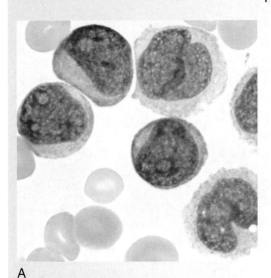

A

Figure 16-6A Peripheral blood (×1000).

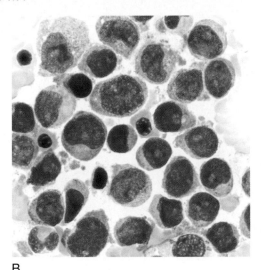

B

Figure 16-6B Bone marrow (×500).

Peripheral Blood: Myeloblasts and other immature myeloid cells, monocytoid cells, thrombocytopenia, ±Auer rods

Bone Marrow: Myeloblasts, promyelocytes, and other myeloid precursors comprise between 30% and 80% NEC, monocytic component >20%, MPX >3% (see Figure 21-1A), α–naphthyl butyrate esterase (NBE)-positive (see Figure 21-1C), ±Auer rods

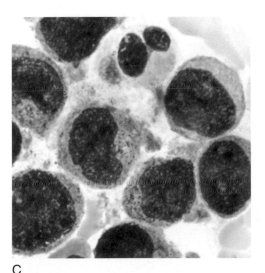

C

Figure 16-6C Bone marrow (×1000).

ACUTE MYELOMONOCYTIC LEUKEMIA WITH EOSINOPHILIA
FAB M4 Eo

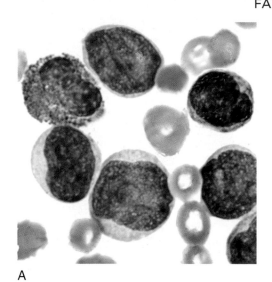

A

Figure 16-7A Peripheral blood (×1000).

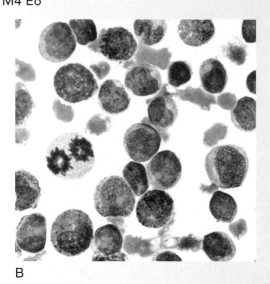

B

Figure 16-7B Bone marrow (×500).

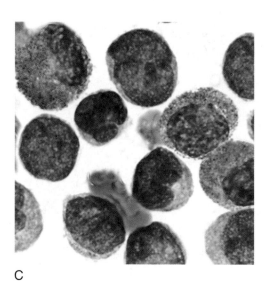

C

Figure 16-7C Bone marrow (×1000).

Peripheral Blood: Myeloblasts and other immature myeloid cells, monocytoid cells, thrombocytopenia

Bone Marrow: Myeloblasts, promyelocytes, and other myeloid precursors comprise between 30% and 80% NEC, monocytic component >20%, MPX positive in >3% of cells (see Figure 21-1A), NBE-positive (see Figure 21-1C), ±Auer rods, >5% eosinophils; may be hybrid with basophilic granules

ACUTE MONOCYTIC LEUKEMIA, POORLY DIFFERENTIATED
FAB M5a

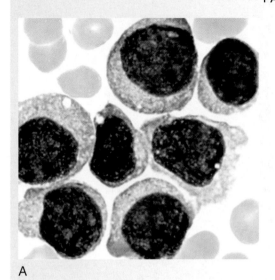

A

Figure 16-8A Peripheral blood (×1000).

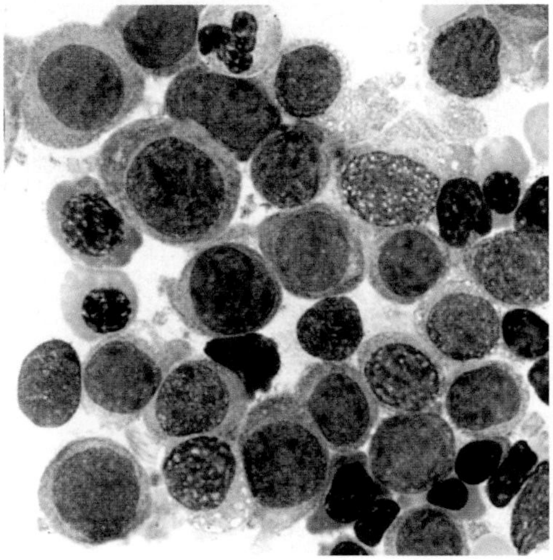

Figure 16-8B Bone marrow (×500).

B

Peripheral Blood: Blasts, thrombocytopenia
Bone Marrow: >20% blasts, >80% have
  monocytic morphology, granulocytic
  component <20%, MPX <3% positive (see
  Figure 21-1A), NBE-positive (see
  Figure 21-1C)

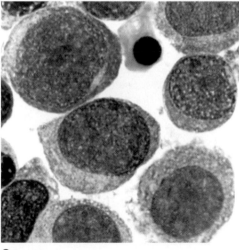

C

Figure 16-8C Bone marrow (×1000).

ACUTE MONOCYTIC LEUKEMIA, WELL-DIFFERENTIATED
FAB M5b

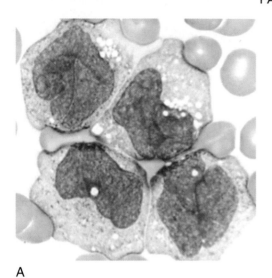

A

Figure 16-9A Peripheral blood (×1000).

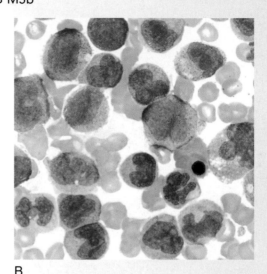

B

Figure 16-9B Bone marrow (×500).

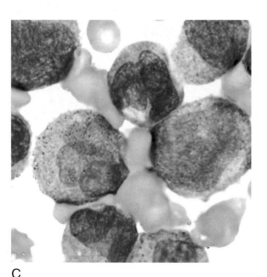

C

Figure 16-9C Bone marrow (×1000).

Peripheral Blood: Blasts, monocytoid cells, thrombocytopenia

Bone Marrow: Monocytic component >80%, monoblasts <80% with promonocytes and monocytes, MPX <3% positive (see Figure 21-1A), NBE-positive (see Figure 21-1C)

ACUTE ERYTHROLEUKEMIA
FAB M6

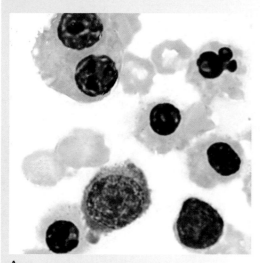

A

Figure 16-10A Peripheral blood (×1000).

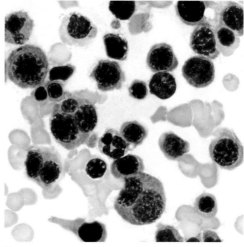

B

Figure 16-10B Bone marrow (×500).

Peripheral Blood: Thrombocytopenia; dimorphic, dichromic erythroid population; basophilic stippling; nucleated erythrocytes; ±blasts

Bone Marrow: ≥20% blasts NEC, ≥50% blasts ANC, bizarre erythroid precursors, periodic acid-Schiff (PAS)-positive with "chunky" or block positivity (see Figure 21-1D)

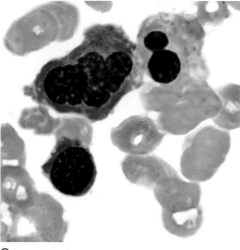

C

Figure 16-10C Bone marrow (×1000).

ACUTE MEGAKARYOCYTIC LEUKEMIA
FAB M7

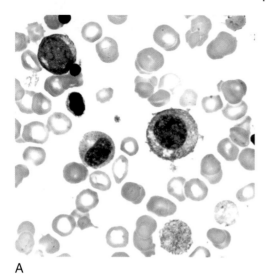

A

Figure 16-11A Peripheral blood (×500).

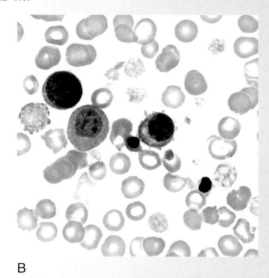

B

Figure 16-11B Peripheral blood (×500).

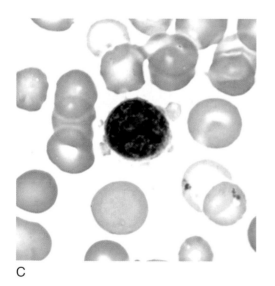

C

Figure 16-11C Peripheral blood (×1000).

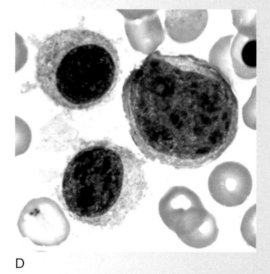

D

Figure 16-11D Peripheral blood (×1000).

Peripheral Blood: ±Micromegakaryocytes, pleomorphic blasts, blasts with agranular cytoplasm, platelet count may be normal or elevated

Bone Marrow: Usually results in a dry tap; >20% blasts ANC, >30% of those being megakaryoblasts; heterogeneous in size, high N/C ratio; may have abundant budding cytoplasm; MPX/SBB-negative (see Figures 21-1A and 21-1B); positive for platelet peroxidase by EM; immunostain for Factor VIII-positive (see Figure 21-4)

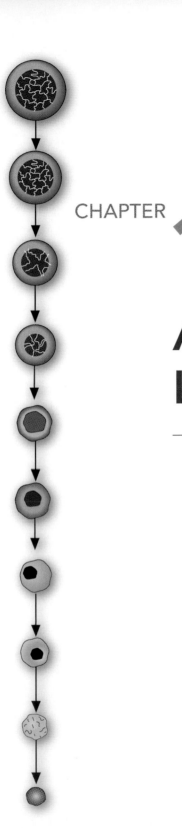

CHAPTER

17

Acute Lymphoid Leukemia

Lymphocytic leukemias are not classified morphologically but by a combination of cytogenetic profiles, genotype, and immunophenotype. The previous FAB lymphoid L1 and L2 morphologies may be either pre-B or pre-T. FAB L3 leukemia is classified by the World Health Organization (WHO) as a mature neoplasm (Burkitt lymphoma) (see Figure 20-8).

BOX 17-1 Acute Lymphoid Leukemias

FAB classification
- ALL L1
- ALL L2
- ALL L3 (no longer considered an acute leukemia; see Chapter 20)

WHO classification
- Precursor B lymphoblastic leukemia/lymphoma (Pre-B)
- Precursor T lymphoblastic leukemia/lymphoma (Pre-T)

ALL, Acute lymphoid leukemia.

ACUTE LYMPHOID LEUKEMIA
Small Lymphoblasts

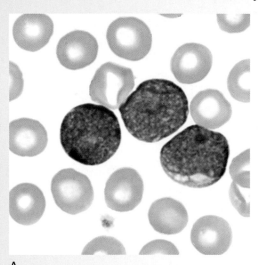

A

Figure 17-1A Peripheral blood (×1000).

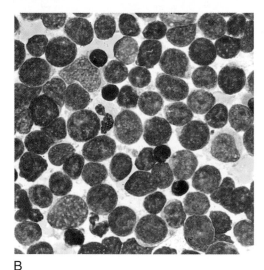

B

Figure 17-1B Bone marrow (×500).

Peripheral Blood: ±Blasts, small blasts with scant blue cytoplasm and round nucleoli, thrombocytopenia

Bone Marrow: >20% blasts; homogeneous population, myeloperoxidase (MPX)-negative (see Figure 21-1A), Sudan Black B (SBB)-negative (see Figure 21-1B), periodic acid-Schiff (PAS)—variable, often positive (see Figure 21-1D)

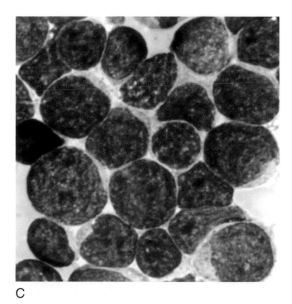

C

Figure 17-1C Bone marrow (×1000).

ACUTE LYMPHOID LEUKEMIA
Large Lymphoblasts

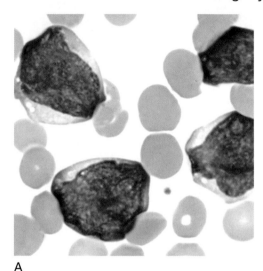

A

Figure 17-2A Peripheral blood (×1000).

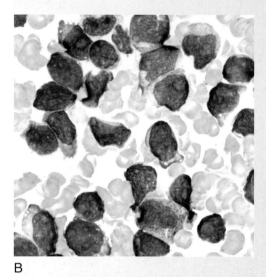

B

Figure 17-2B Bone marrow (×500).

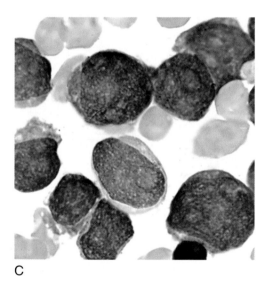

C

Figure 17-2C Bone marrow (×1000).

Peripheral Blood: Blasts—2 to 3 times the size of a resting lymphocyte, moderate cytoplasm, irregular nuclear membrane, prominent nucleoli, thrombocytopenia, morphologically difficult to distinguish from acute myeloid leukemia

Bone Marrow: >20% blasts, heterogeneous population, myeloperoxidase (MPX)-negative (see Figure 21-1A), Sudan Black B (SBB)-negative (see Figure 21-1B), periodic acid-Schiff (PAS)—variable, often positive (see Figure 21-1D)

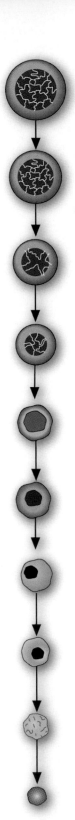

CHAPTER

18

Myeloproliferative Disorders

BOX 18-1 Myeloproliferative Syndromes

FAB classification
- Polycythemia vera
- Essential thrombocythemia
- Myelofibrosis
- CML

WHO classification
- Polycythemia vera
- Essential thrombocythemia
- Chronic idiopathic myelofibrosis
- Chronic myelogenous leukemia, Philadelphia chromosome positive (ph)[t(9;22)(q34q11),BCR/ABL]
- Chronic neutrophilic leukemia
- Chronic eosinophilic leukemia/hypereosinophilic syndrome

Philadelphia chromosome negative CML, chronic myelomonocytic leukemia, and juvenile myelomonocytic leukemia belong to a new WHO classification of myelodysplastic/myeloproliferative disorders.

FAB, French-American-British; *CML,* chronic myelogenous leukemia; *WHO,* World Health Organization.

CHRONIC MYELOGENOUS LEUKEMIA (CML)

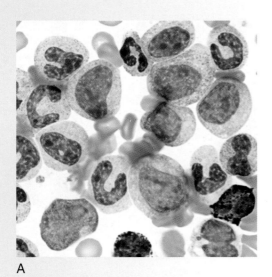

A

Figure 18-1A Peripheral blood (original ×1000).

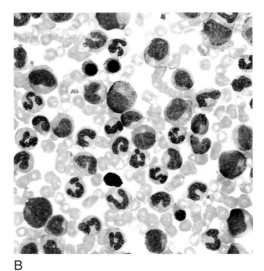

B

Figure 18-1B Bone marrow (original ×500).

Peripheral Blood: Marked leukocytosis (usually >50.0 × 10⁹/L)
- Spectrum of myeloid cells with a predominance of myelocytes and polymorphonuclear neutrophils
- Myeloblasts and promyelocytes: 1%-5%
- ± Pseudo-Pelger-Huët cells
- Eosinophilia and/or basophilia
- Monocytosis
    - Platelets: Normal to increased
    - ± Circulating micromegakaryocytes
    - Leukocyte alkaline phosphatase (LAP): Markedly decreased (see Figure 21-3)

Bone Marrow: Hypercellular with expansion of granulocyte pool, myeloid:erythroid (M:E) ratio increased ≥10:1, myeloblasts and promyelocytes <30%, megakaryocytes—normal to increased; may be immature and/or atypical

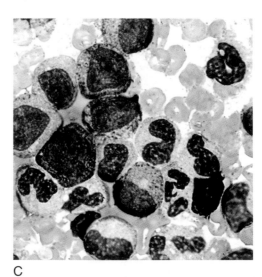

C

Figure 18-1C Bone marrow (original ×1000).

POLYCYTHEMIA VERA (PV)

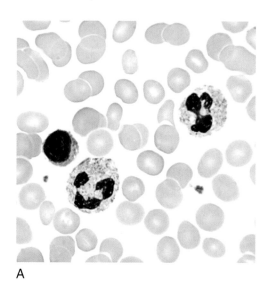

A

Figure 18-2A Peripheral blood (original ×1000).

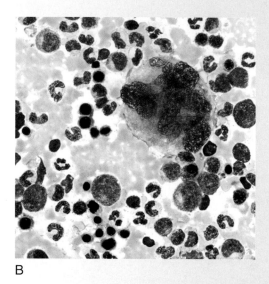

B

Figure 18-2B Bone marrow (original ×500).

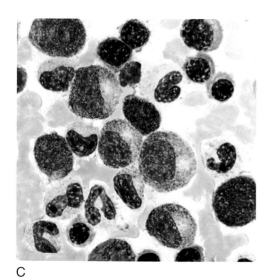

C

Figure 18-2C Bone marrow (original ×1000).

Peripheral blood: Absolute erythrocytosis
Moderate leukocytosis (12.0 to 25.0 × 10⁹/L)
- Neutrophilia with few metamyelocytes, rare myelocytes
- Promyelocytes and myeloblasts extremely rare
- ± Eosinophilia and/or basophilia
    - Thrombocytosis
    - LAP: Normal or increased

Bone Marrow: Hypercellular with panhyperplasia, M:E ratio—usually normal, megakaryocytes may be abnormal in size and morphology

NOTE: The diagnosis of polycythemia vera is not made on morphology but on the basis of an elevated erythrocyte mass and normal oxygen saturation.

ESSENTIAL THROMBOCYTHEMIA (ET)

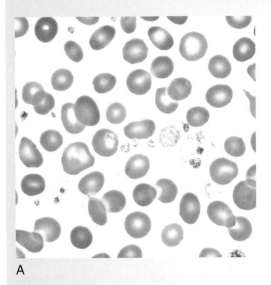

A

Figure 18-3A Peripheral blood (original ×1000).

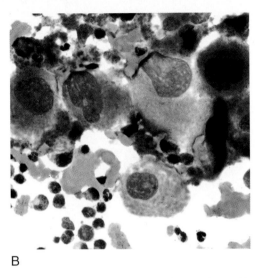

B

Figure 18-3B Bone marrow (original ×500).

Peripheral Blood: Marked thrombocytosis
(>600.0 × 10⁹/L)
- Abnormal platelet morphology (variations
in size, shape, and granulation); often
present in clusters
    - ±Leukocytosis: Neutrophilia with
    bands and metamyelocytes
    - LAP: Normal or increased
    (see Figure 21-3)

Bone Marrow: Hypercellular with expansion
of the megakaryocyte pool
- Large megakaryocytes with abundant
cytoplasm may exhibit hyperlobulation
    - Mild granulocytic hyperplasia
    - Mild erythrocytic hyperplasia

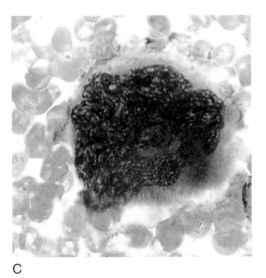

C

Figure 18-3C Bone marrow (original ×1000).

MYELOFIBROSIS WITH MYELOID METAPLASIA (MMM)
Agnogenic Myeloid Metaplasia (AMM)

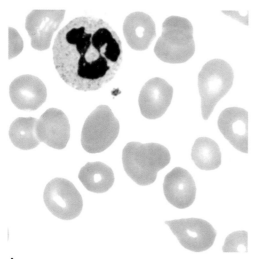

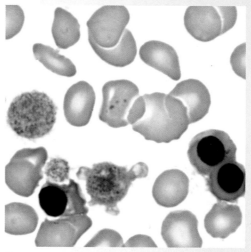

A

B

Figure 18-4A Peripheral blood (×1000) (subtle changes).

Figure 18-4B Peripheral blood (×1000) (more advanced case).

MILD ERYTHROCYTIC HYPERPLASIA
Peripheral Blood:
Erythrocytes:
- Tear drop cells common, nucleated erythrocytes, polychromasia
Leukocytes:
- Normal, increased, or decreased
- Immature granulocytes
- <5% blasts
- ±Basophilia and eosinophilia
- Morphological abnormalities
  LAP: Normal, increased, or decreased
Platelets:
- Low, normal, or increased
- Giant bizarre shapes
- Abnormal granulation
- ±Circulating megakaryocytes

Bone Marrow: Aspiration attempts often result in a dry tap; biopsies exhibit marked fibrosis with islands of hematopoietic activity

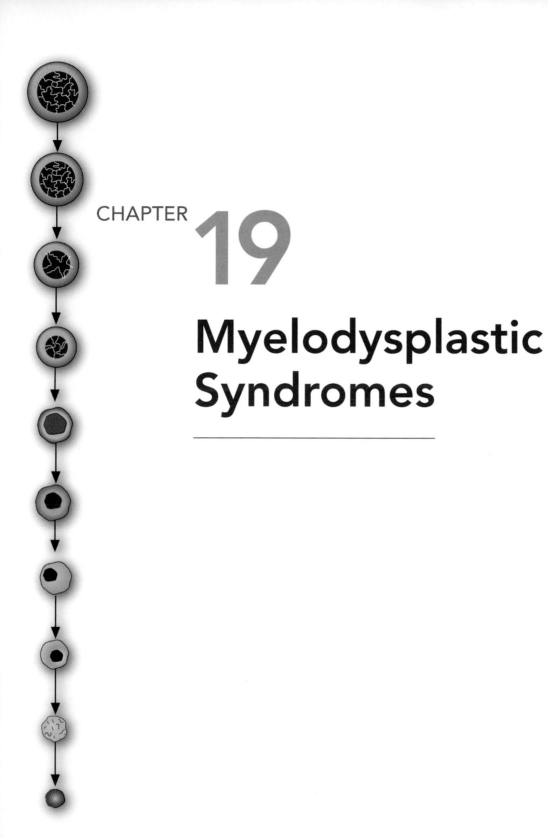

19

Myelodysplastic Syndromes

Myelodysplastic syndromes (MDSs) are acquired clonal hematological disorders characterized by progressive cytopenias in peripheral blood, reflecting maturation defects in erythrocytes, leukocytes, and/or platelets.

BOX 19-1 Myelodysplastic Syndromes

French-American-British (FAB) Classification
- Refractory anemia (RA)
- Refractory anemia with ringed sideroblasts (RARS)
- Refractory anemia with excess blasts (RAEB)
- Refractory anemia with excess blasts in transformation (RAEB-t)
- Chronic myelomonocytic leukemia (CMML)*

World Health Organization (WHO) Classification
- Refractory anemia (RA)
- Refractory cytopenia with multi-lineage dysplasia (RCMD)
- Refractory anemia with excess blasts (RAEB)
- $5q^-$ syndrome
- Myelodysplastic syndrome, unclassified

---

*FAB chronic myelomonocytic leukemia has become part of the new WHO classification of myelodysplastic/myeloproliferative disorders.

DYSERYTHROPOIESIS

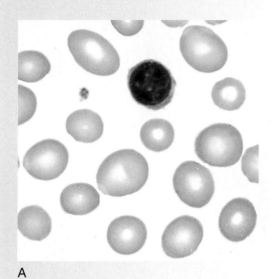

A

Figure 19-1A Oval macrocytes (PB ×1000).

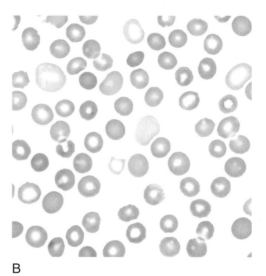

B

Figure 19-1B Dimorphic erythrocyte population (PB ×500).

Evidence of dyserythropoiesis (Figures 19-1A to 19-1I) may include any or all of the following: oval macrocytes, hypochromic microcytes, dimorphic erythrocyte population, erythrocyte precursors with >1 nucleus, abnormal nuclear shapes, nuclear bridging, uneven cytoplasmic staining, and/or ringed sideroblasts

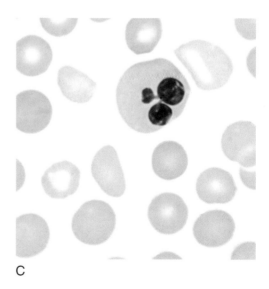

C

Figure 19-1C Nucleated erythrocyte with abnormal nuclear shape (PB ×1000).

All photomicrographs are ×1000 with Wright–Giemsa stain unless stated otherwise.

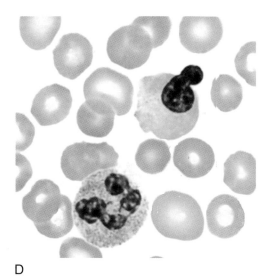

D

Figure 19-1D Erythrocyte precursor with partial loss of nucleus (PB ×1000).

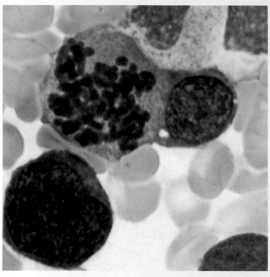

E

Figure 19-1E Erythrocyte precursor with abnormal nuclear shape (bilobed, with one nucleus in mitosis, demonstrating asynchrony) (BM ×1000).

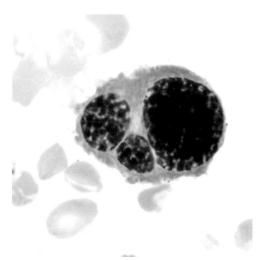

F

Figure 19-1F Erythrocyte precursor with three uneven nuclei (BM ×1000).

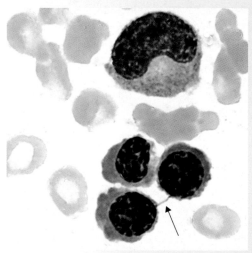

G

Figure 19-1G Erythrocyte precursor with nuclear bridging (BM ×1000).

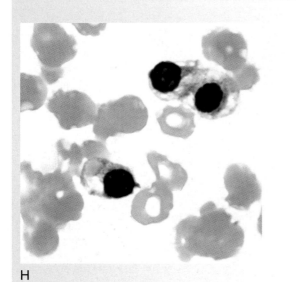

H

Figure 19-1H Erythrocyte precursors with uneven cytoplasmic staining (BM ×1000).

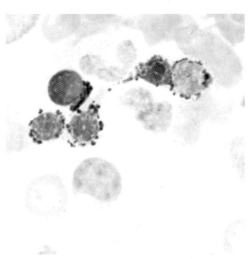

I

Figure 19-1I Ringed sideroblasts (iron stain, BM ×1000).

DYSMYELOPOIESIS

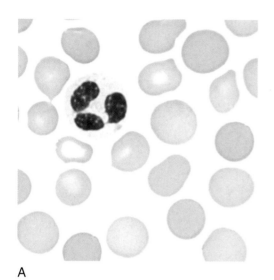

A

Figure 19-2A Abnormal granulation, agranular polymorphonuclear neutrophil.

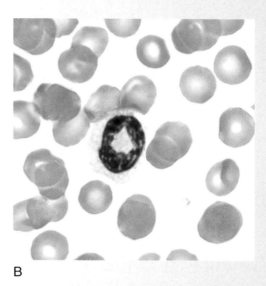

B

Figure 19-2B Abnormal nuclear shapes, neutrophil with circular (donut) nucleus.

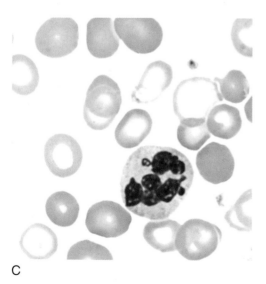

C

Figure 19-2C Abnormal nuclear shapes, neutrophil with hypersegmented nucleus; also exhibits degranulation.

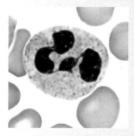

Normal neutrophil for comparison.

Evidence of dysmyelopoiesis (Figures 19-2A to 19-2F) may include any or all of the following: abnormal granulation, abnormal nuclear shapes, persistent basophilic cytoplasm, and/or uneven cytoplasmic staining

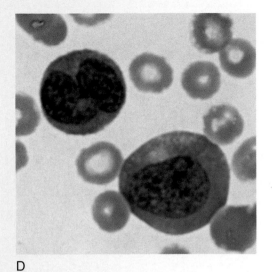

D

Figure 19-2D Persistent basophilic cytoplasm.

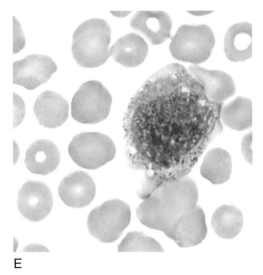

E

Figure 19-2E Uneven cytoplasmic staining with uneven granulation.

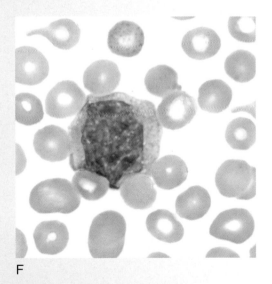

F

Figure 19-2F Uneven cytoplasmic staining.

DYSMEGAKARYOPOIESIS

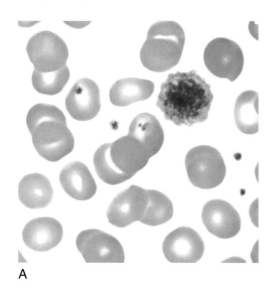

A

Figure 19-3A Giant platelet.

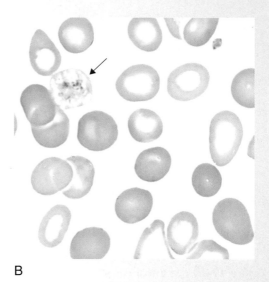

B

Figure 19-3B Platelet with abnormal granulation.

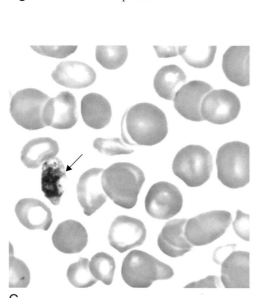

C

Figure 19-3C Platelet with abnormal granulation.

Evidence of dysmegakaryopoiesis (Figures 19-3A to 19-3H) may include any or all of the following: giant platelets, platelets with abnormal granulation, circulating micromegakaryocytes, large mononuclear megakaryocytes, abnormal nuclear shapes

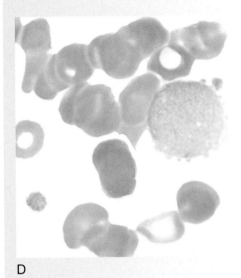

D

Figure 19-3D Megakaryocyte fragment.

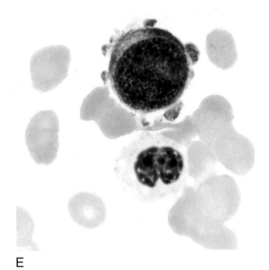

E

Figure 19-3E Circulating micromegakaryocyte.

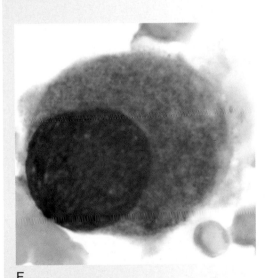

F

Figure 19-3F Large mononuclear megakaryocyte (BM ×1000).

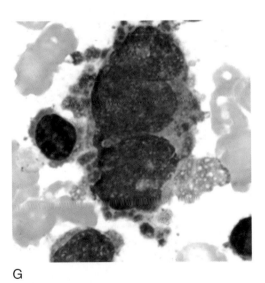

G

Figure 19-3G Abnormal nuclear shape, uneven number of nuclei (BM ×1000).

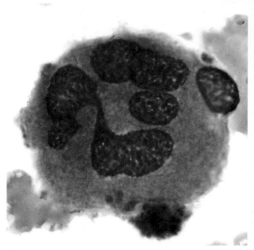

H

Figure 19-3H Abnormal nuclear shapes, separate nuclei (BM, original magnification ×1000).

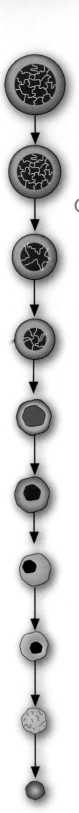

CHAPTER

20

Malignant Lymphoproliferative Disorders

Malignant lymphoproliferative disorders frequently are derived from a single clone of cells. Although this group of diseases involves lymphocytes, the morphological presentation is variable. The integration of clinical and morphological disease features with immunophenotyping and cytogenetic and molecular studies is necessary for appropriate recognition and classification. Only representative samples are included in this atlas.

NOTE: Any absolute lymphocytosis in an adult should be investigated.

PROLYMPHOCYTIC LEUKEMIA (PLL)

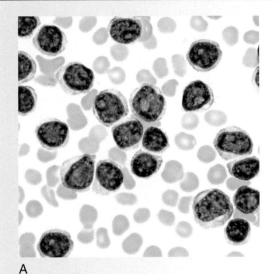

A

Figure 20-1A Peripheral blood (PB ×500).

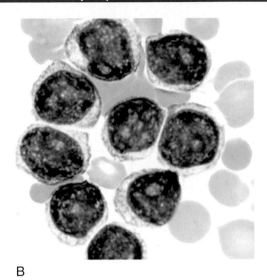

B

Figure 20-1B (PB ×1000).

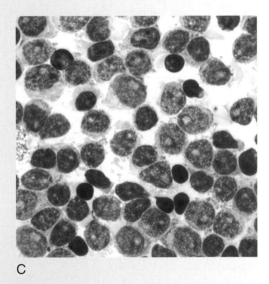

C

Figure 20-1C Bone marrow (BM ×500).

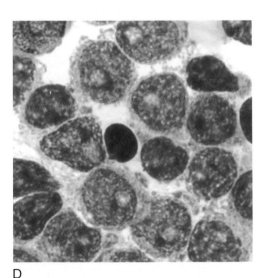

D

Figure 20-1D (BM ×1000).

Peripheral Blood: Absolute lymphocytosis, usually >100 × 10^9/L, relatively large cells having one prominent nucleolus, chromatin structure intermediate between that of a blast and a mature lymphocyte, relatively uniform within a given patient, anemia, thrombocytopenia

Bone Marrow: Predominantly prolymphocytes with very few residual hematopoietic cells

CHRONIC LYMPHOCYTIC LEUKEMIA (CLL)

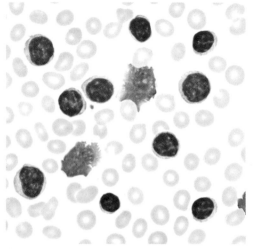

A

Figure 20-2A (PB ×500).

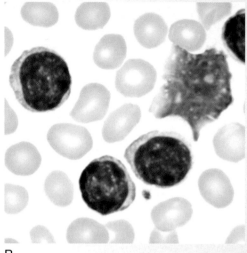

B

Figure 20-2B (PB ×1000).

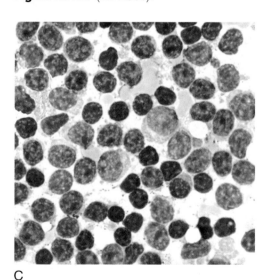

C

Figure 20-2C (BM ×500).

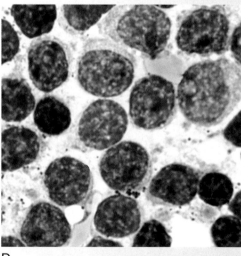

D

Figure 20-2D (BM ×1000).

Peripheral Blood: Absolute sustained lymphocytosis (10 to 150 × 10^9/L); homogeneous appearance within a given patient; mature-appearing lymphocytes with round nuclei and block-type chromatin; cytoplasm scant or moderate; lymphocytes more fragile than normal, leading to "smudge" cells; normocytic normochromic anemia, which increases with disease progression; approximately 10% of patients develop a hemolytic anemia; thrombocytopenia with disease progression

Bone Marrow: ≥30% lymphocytes

HAIRY CELL LEUKEMIA (HCL)

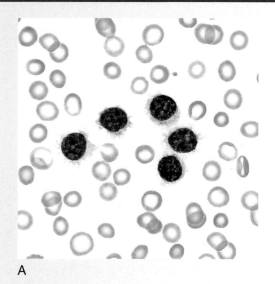

A

Figure 20-3A (PB ×500).

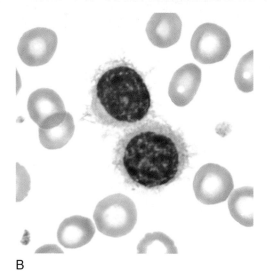

B

Figure 20-3B (PB ×1000).

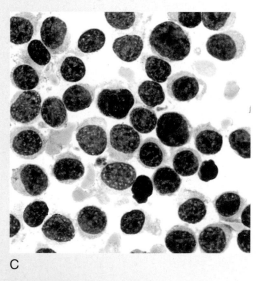

C

Figure 20-3C (BM ×500).

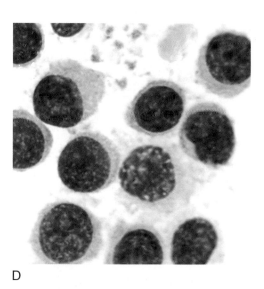

D

Figure 20-3D (BM ×1000).

Peripheral Blood: Pancytopenia, reniform to oval nuclei with diffuse homogeneous chromatin, may have a single nucleolus, cytoplasm irregular and gray-blue with delicate hairlike cytoplasmic projections

Bone Marrow: Aspirate difficult to obtain due to marrow fibrosis (dry tap), cells more easily distinguished by phase or electron microscopy, cells positive by the tartrate-resistant acid phosphatase (TRAP) stain (see Figure 21-2)

WALDENSTRÖM MACROGLOBULINEMIA

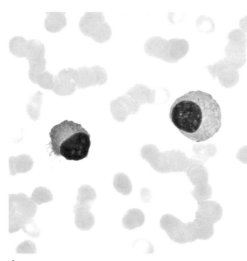

A

Figure 20-4A (PB ×500).

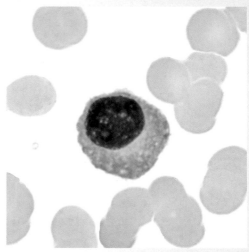

B

Figure 20-4B (PB ×1000).

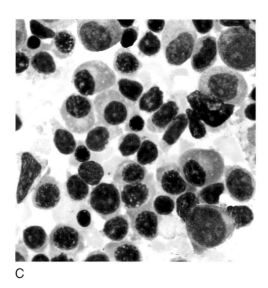

C

Figure 20-4C (BM ×500).

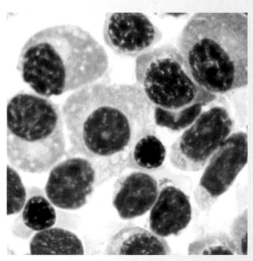

D

Figure 20-4D (BM ×1000).

Peripheral Blood: Leukocyte count usually normal, rare plasmacytoid cell or plasma cell, normocytic normochromic anemia with rouleaux, normal to decreased platelet numbers

NOTE: The background of Wright-stained blood smears may be blue owing to abnormal amounts of immunoglobulin.

Bone Marrow: Hypercellular with plasmacytoid infiltrates

NOTE: This disease may be distinguished from multiple myeloma and heavy chain disease by immunoelectrophoresis.

MULTIPLE MYELOMA

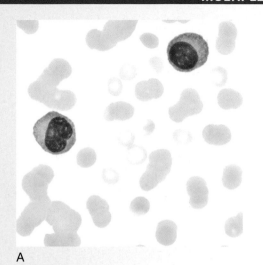

A

Figure 20-5A (PB ×500).

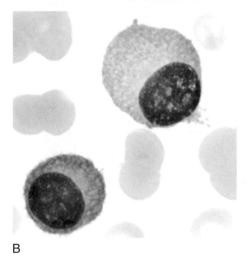

B

Figure 20-5B (PB ×1000).

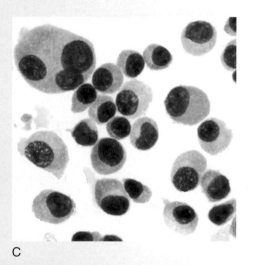

C

Figure 20-5C (BM ×500).

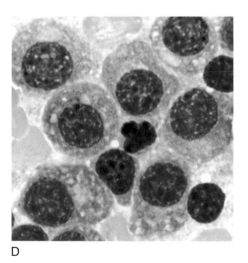

D

Figure 20-5D (BM ×1000).

Peripheral Blood: Possible neutropenia, rare abnormal circulating plasma cell, normocytic normochromic anemia, rouleaux, platelet count normal to decreased. If greater than 2×10^9/L plasma cells are circulating in the peripheral blood, plasma-cell leukemia is present.

NOTE: The background of Wright-stained blood smears may be blue owing to abnormal amounts of immunoglobulin.

Bone Marrow: >10% abnormal plasma cells, often >30%; larger than normal plasma cell with increased N/C ratio; immature in appearance; abnormal nuclear chromatin; ±nucleoli, nucleus may be centrally located; ±multinucleated; possible loss of nuclear hof; cytoplasm may be pale blue or dark; cytoplasm may contain immunoglobulin inclusions

NOTE: This disease may be distinguished from Waldenström macroglobulinemia and heavy chain disease by immunoelectrophoresis.

NON-HODGKIN LYMPHOMAS

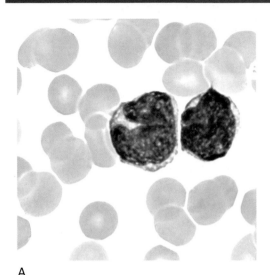

A

Figure 20-6A (PB ×1000).

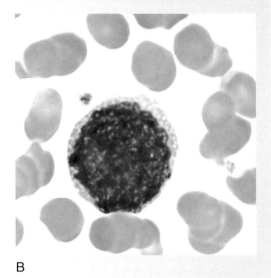

B

Figure 20-6B (PB ×1000).

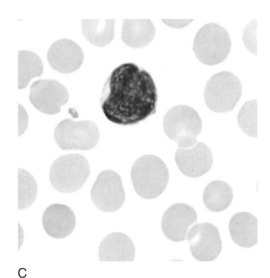

C

Figure 20-6C (PB ×1000).

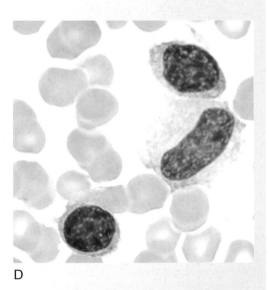

D

Figure 20-6D (PB ×1000).

Peripheral Blood: A variety of lymphoma cells has been illustrated because occasionally lymphoma cells are found in the peripheral blood. The diagnosis of lymphoma is determined by lymph node biopsy, immunophenotyping, and cytogenetics.

Bone Marrow: NA

T-CELL LEUKEMIA/LYMPHOMA

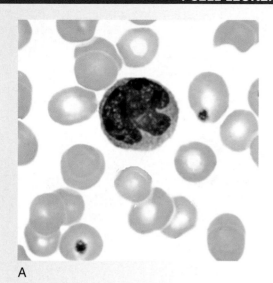

A

Figure 20-7A T-cell lymphoma (PB ×1000).

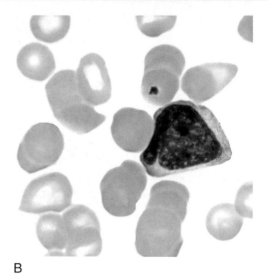

B

Figure 20-7B T-cell lymphoma (PB ×1000).

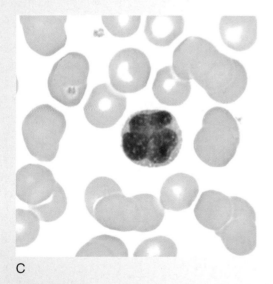

C

Figure 20-7C T-cell lymphoma (PB ×1000).

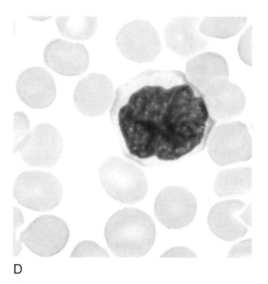

D

Figure 20-7D Sézary cell (PB ×1000).

Peripheral Blood: Leukocytosis. Size of cell and shape of nucleus vary; multilobed nucleus may resemble a cloverleaf. Chromatin is moderately condensed; nucleoli are inconspicuous. Sézary cells in the peripheral blood are morphologically altered T cells and represent the cutaneous T-cell lymphoma mycosis fungoides, which involves the skin.

Bone Marrow: NA

BURKITT LEUKEMIA/LYMPHOMA

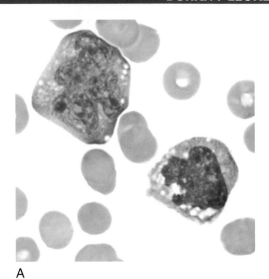

A

Figure 20-8A (PB ×1000).

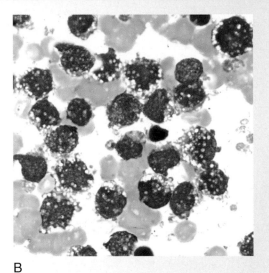

B

Figure 20-8B (BM ×500).

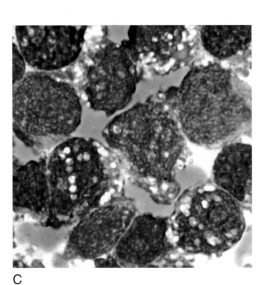

C

Figure 20-8C (BM ×1000).

Peripheral Blood: Medium to large size cells with dark blue cytoplasm, vacuoles in cytoplasm, 3-5 nucleoli, thrombocytopenia

Bone Marrow: Monotonous pattern of deeply basophilic cells with vacuoles

Burkitt leukemia/lymphoma was classified in the French–American–British system as L3 acute leukemia. The cells are actually mature B cells, thus Burkitt lymphoma is classified by the WHO as a mature B-cell neoplasm.

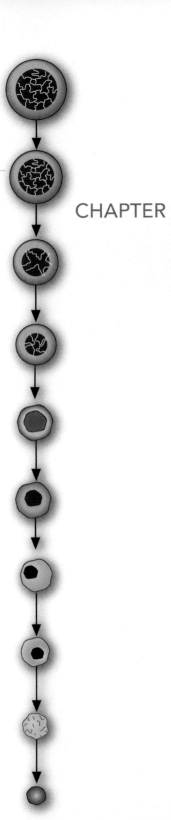

CHAPTER

21

Cytochemical Stains

Figure 21-1 demonstrates stains that are used primarily to differentiate acute leukemias. Results are summarized in Table 21-1.

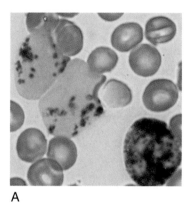

A

Figure 21-1A Myeloperoxidase (MPX) (Bone marrow [BM] × 1000).

Stains granules containing peroxidase, that is, primary granules in neutrophils and granules in eosinophils and monocytes.

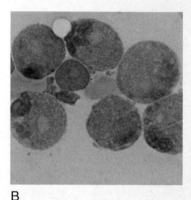

B

Figure 21-1B Sudan Black B (SBB) (BM × 1000).

Stains lipids, including neutral fat, phospholipids, and sterols. Parallels myeloperoxidase reaction.

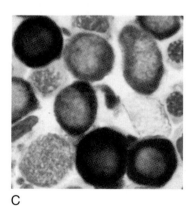

C

Figure 21-1C α-Naphthyl butyrate esterase (NBE) (BM ×1000).

Esterase hydrolyzes an ester. Diffusely positive in monocytes, and negative or focally positive in the neutrophil series.

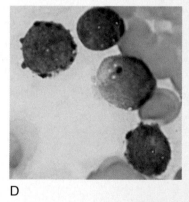

D

Figure 21-1D Periodic acid–Schiff (PAS) (BM × 1000).

Stains carbohydrates, primarily glycogen. Block positivity is associated with acute lymphoblastic leukemia and early precursors of erythroleukemia (FAB M6). Later precursors show diffuse positivity.

TABLE 21-1 Simplified Acute Leukemia Reaction Chart

Condition	Cytochemical Stain*						
	MPX	**SBB**	**NASDA**	**ANBE**	**ANAE**	**PAS**	**Factor VIII**
ALL	−	−	−	−/+ (focal)	−/+ (focal)	Varied	−
AML	+	+	+	−	−	Varied	−
AMML	+	+	+	+ (diffuse)	+ (diffuse)	Varied	−
AmoL	−	−	−	+ (diffuse)	+ (diffuse)	Varied	−
Erythroleukemia	*	*	*	−	−	Blocky in pronormoblasts	−
Megakaryocytic	−	−	−	−	+ (localized)	−/+ (localized)	+

From Rodak BF, Fritsma GF, Doig K: *Hematology: clinical principles and applications*, ed 3, St Louis, 2007, Saunders. *MPX*, Myeloperoxidase; *SBB*, Sudan black B; *NASDA*, naphthol AS-D chloroacetate esterase; *ANBE*, α-naphthyl butyrate esterase; *ANAE*, α-naphthyl acetate esterase; *PAS*, periodic acid–Schiff; *ALL*, acute lymphocytic leukemia; *AML*, acute myeloid leukemia; *AMML*, acute myelomonocytic leukemia; *AmoL*, acute monocytic leukemia.
* Positive in myeloblasts; negative in normoblasts.

TARTRATE-RESISTANT LEUKOCYTE ACID PHOSPHATE (TRAP)

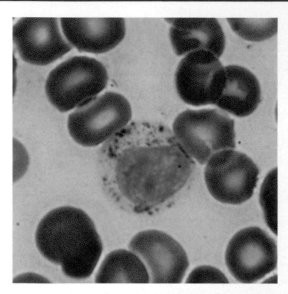

Figure 21-2 Tartrate–resistant leukocyte acid phosphatase (TRAP).

Positive in most cases of hairy cell leukemia. Those cells contain acid phosphatase and remain positive after the addition of L(+)-tartaric acid.

LEUKOCYTE ALKALINE PHOSPHATASE (LAP)

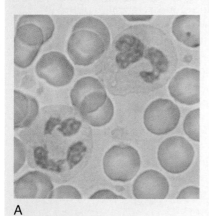

A

Figure 21-3A Leukocyte alkaline phosphatase (LAP)–negative reaction (0) (PB × 1000).

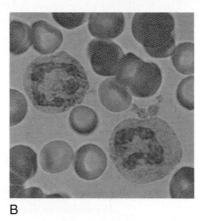

B

Figure 21-3B LAP (1+) (PB × 1000).

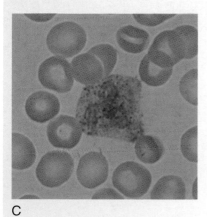

C

Figure 21-3C LAP (2+) (PB × 1000).

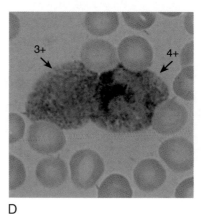

D

Figure 21-3D LAP (3+, 4+) (PB × 1000).

Leukocyte alkaline phosphatase (LAP) is an enzyme found in secondary granules of neutrophils. LAP activity is scored from 0 to 4+ in the mature polymorphonuclear neutrophils and bands. One hundred cells are scored and results are added together for the LAP score. A normal score is approximately 20 to 100. Low (<20) scores may be found in untreated chronic myeloid leukemia, paroxysmal nocturnal hemoglobinuria, sideroblastic anemia, and myelodysplastic syndromes. Higher scores may be found in leukemoid reactions, polycythemia vera, and the third trimester of pregnancy. See Table 21-2.

TABLE 21-2 Results of Leukocyte Alkaline Phosphatase Stain

Finding	Score
Normal	20-100
Chronic myelogenous leukemia	<13
Leukemoid reaction	>100
Polycythemia vera	100-200
Secondary polycythemia	20-100

IMMUNOPEROXIDASE

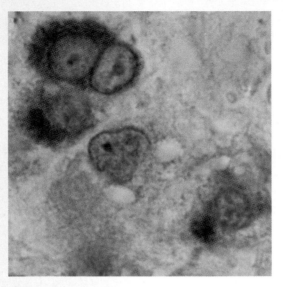

Figure 21-4 Immunoperoxidase reaction for Factor VIII (BM ×1000).

This is an example of an immunohistochemical stain in which the antigen-antibody bond is visualized by tagging the antibody with an indicator, such as an enzyme or a fluorochrome.

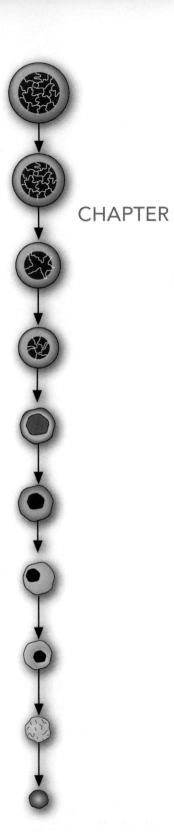

22

Microorganisms

PLASMODIUM SPECIES

The following are representative examples of the developmental stages of malaria that can be seen in the peripheral blood. Detailed criteria for identification of species may be found in a parasitology text.

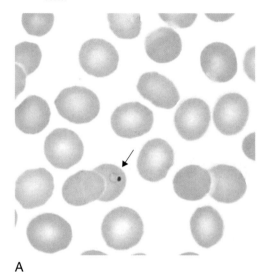

A

Figure 22-1A *Plasmodium* species (peripheral blood [PB] ×1000).

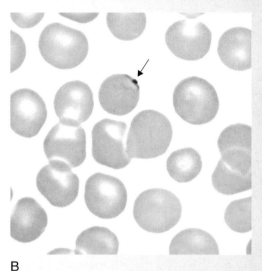

B

Figure 22-1B *Appliqué form (PB ×1000).*

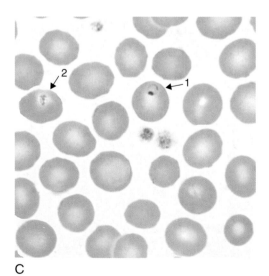

C

Figure 22-1C Platelet versus malaria: *1*, malaria, *2*, platelet (PB ×1000).

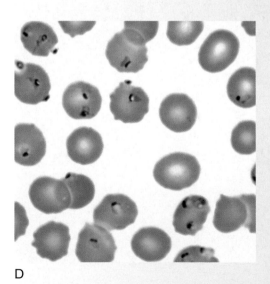

D

Figure 22-1D *Plasmodium* species—multiple rings as often seen in *P. falciparum* (PB ×1000).

PLASMODIUM SPECIES

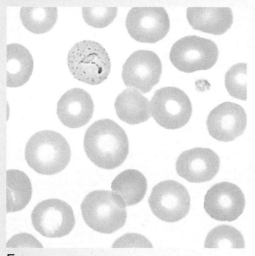

E

Figure 22-1E *Plasmodium* species (PB ×1000).

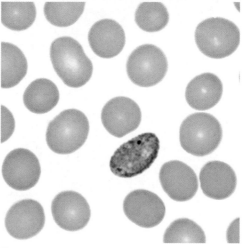

F

Figure 22-1F *Plasmodium* species (PB ×1000).

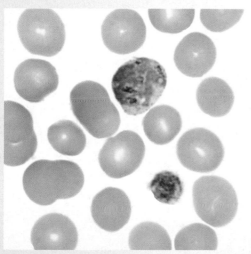

G

Figure 22-1G *Plasmodium* species (PB ×1000).

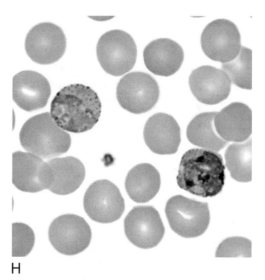

H

Figure 22-1H *Plasmodium* species (PB ×1000).

BABESIA SPECIES

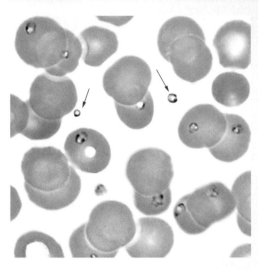

Figure 22-2 *Babesia microti* (PB ×1000).

Babesia species may be confused morphologically with *Plasmodium falciparum*, but lack of pigment, and absence of life cycle stages help differentiate *Babesia* spp. from *P. falciparum*. Another differentiating factor is the presence of extracellular organisms *(arrows)* that may be seen in *Babesia* spp. but not in *P. falciparum*.

LOA LOA

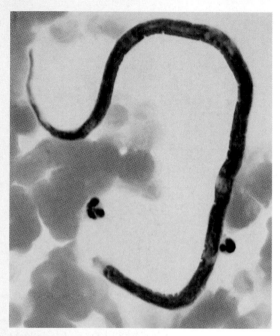

Figure 22-3 *Loa loa*, a microfilaria (PB original magnification ×1000).

Loa loa is a microfilaria. Other microfilariae rarely may be seen in the peripheral blood.

TRYPANOSOMES

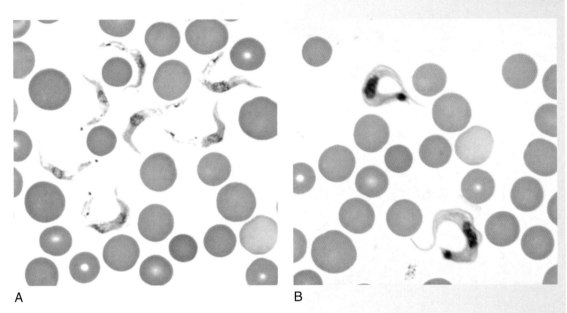

A

B

Figure 22-4A *Trypanosoma gambiense* (Giemsa stain, PB ×1000).

Figure 22-4B *Trypanosoma cruzi* (Giemsa stain, PB ×1000). (From Marler LM, Siders JA, Simpson A et al: *Parasitology image atlas cd-rom,* Indianapolis, Ind, 2003, Indiana Pathology Images).

Trypanosomes are an example of hemoflagellates that may occasionally be encountered in the peripheral blood. Differentiating features may be found in a parasitology text.

FUNGI

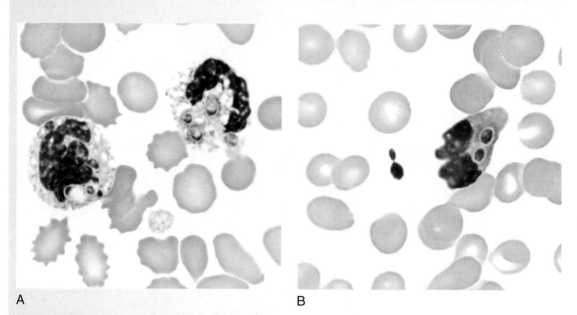

A

B

Figure 22-5A *Histoplasma capsulatum* (PB ×1000).

Figure 22-5B Intracellular and extracellular yeast in peripheral blood of an immunocompromised patient (PB ×1000).

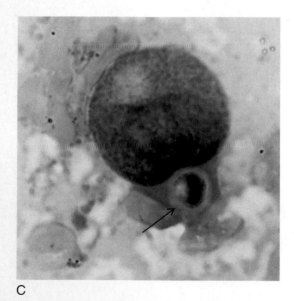

C

Figure 22-5C *Cryptococcus neoformans* (bone marrow ×1000). See also Figure 25-14.

BACTERIA

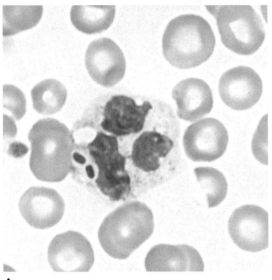

A

Figure 22-6A Coccobacilli engulfed by a leukocyte (PB ×1000).

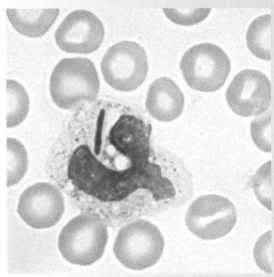

B

Figure 22-6B Bacillus engulfed by a leukocyte (PB ×1000).

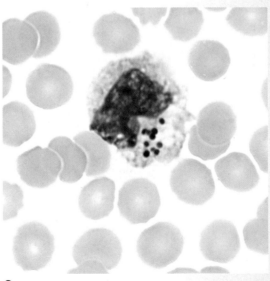

C

Figure 22-6C Cocci engulfed by a monocyte (PB ×1000).

BACTERIA

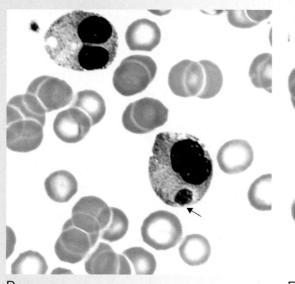

D

Figure 22-6D *Anaplasma phagocytophilum* in a neutrophil (PB ×1000).

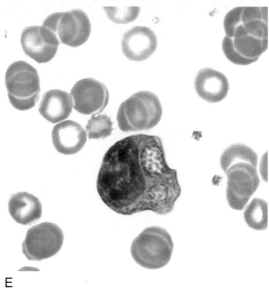

E

Figure 22-6E *Ehrlichia chaffeensis* in a monocyte (PB ×1000). (Courtesy J. Stephen Dumler, MD, Division of Medical Microbiology, The Johns Hopkins Medical Institutions, Baltimore, Md.)

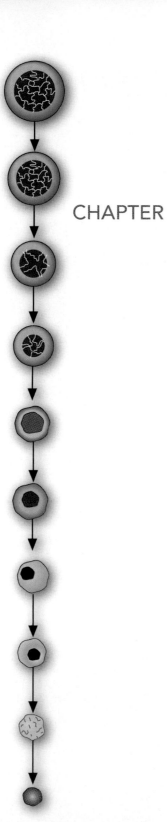

23

Miscellaneous Cells

CELLS OCCASIONALLY SEEN IN BONE MARROW
Fat Cell

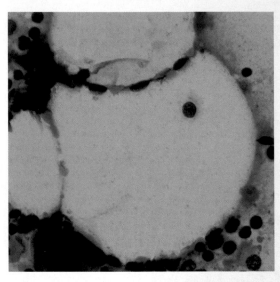

Figure 23-1 Fat cell (bone marrow [BM] ×500).

DESCRIPTION: Large round cell, 50 to 80 μm; cytoplasm filled with one or several large fat vacuoles, colorless to pale blue; nucleus small, round to oval, and eccentric; chromatin coarse; nucleoli seldom seen

Mitosis

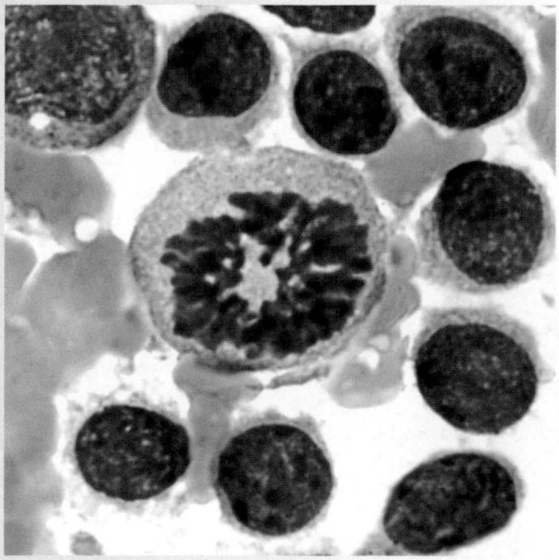

A

Figure 23-2A Mitosis (BM ×1000).

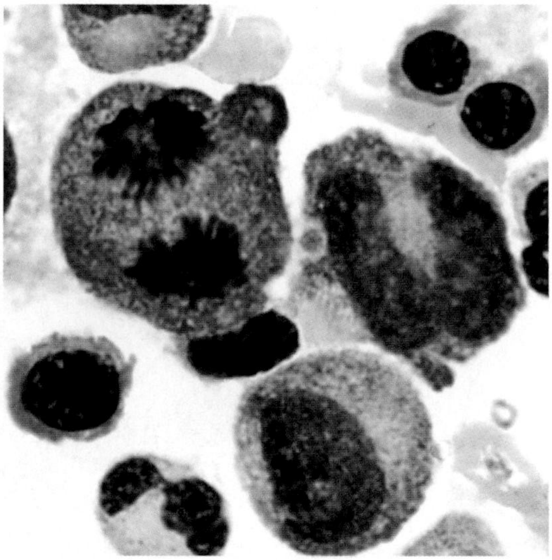

B

Figure 23-2B Mitosis (BM ×1000).

Mitotic figure—a cell that is dividing. Increased numbers may be seen in neoplastic disorders.

Erythroblastic Island

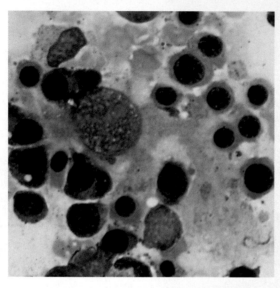

Figure 23-3 Erythroblastic island (nurse cell) (BM ×500).

Iron-laden macrophage surrounded by developing erythroblasts.

Bone Cells

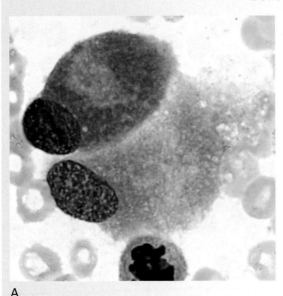

A

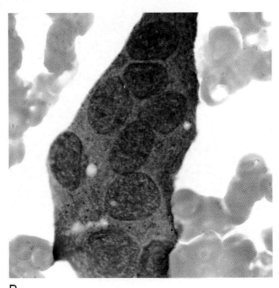

B

Figure 23-4A Osteoblasts (BM original magnification ×1000).

Figure 23-4B Osteoclast (BM original magnification ×1000).

OSTEOBLAST:

Size: 30 µm

Appearance: Comet or tadpole shaped. Single, round, eccentrically placed nucleus, may be partially extruded. Abundant cytoplasm with chromophobic area located away from nucleus. Often appear in groups. Function in synthesis of bone.

OSTEOCLAST:

Size: Very large, greater than 100 µm

Appearance: Cell is irregularly shaped with a ruffled border and is multinucleated. Nuclei are round to oval, separate and distinct, and show very little variation in nuclear size. Nucleoli are usually visible. Cytoplasm may vary from slightly basophilic to very acidophilic. Coarse granules may be present. Osteoclasts function in the resorption of bone.

Metastatic Tumor Cells

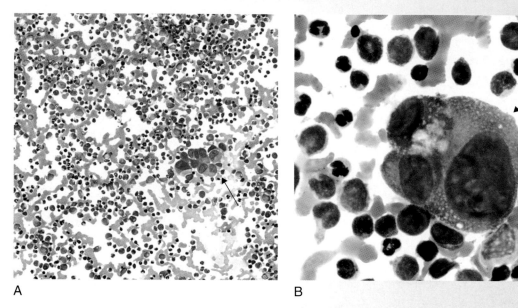

A

B

Figure 23-5A Metastatic tumor (BM ×100).

Figure 23-5B Metastatic tumor (BM ×500).

DESCRIPTION: Tumor cell clusters may be recognized during the 100× scan of bone marrow, especially at or near the edge of the coverslip or glass slide. Characteristics of the tumor cells are more easily observed at 500× magnification. Cells are variable in size and shape within the same tumor clump. Nuclei vary in size and staining characteristics. Nucleoli are usually visible. It is difficult to distinguish one cell from another because of "molding" of cells.

Endothelial Cells

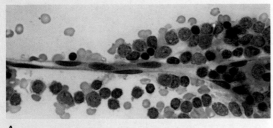

A

Figure 23-6A Endothelial cells (BM original magnification ×500).

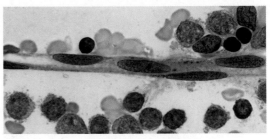

B

Figure 23-6B Endothelial cells (BM original magnification ×1000).

DESCRIPTION: Large elongated cells, 20 to 30 μm. One oval nucleus with dense chromatin; nucleoli not visible. Function is to line blood vessels.

Plasma Cell Variations

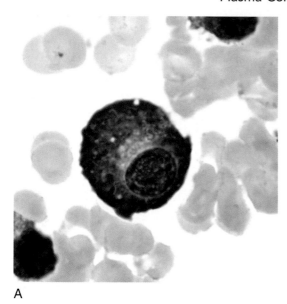

A

Figure 23-7A Plasma cell with red cytoplasm due to high concentration of glycoprotein. Flame cell (BM ×1000).

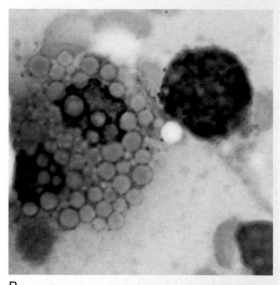

B

Figure 23-7B Plasma cell containing multiple round globules of immunoglobin, which stain pink, colorless, or blue. Mott cell, grape cell, morula cell (BM ×1000).

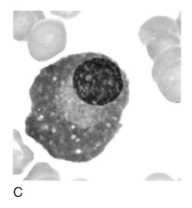

C

Figure 23-7C Normal plasma cell for comparison.

Mast Cell

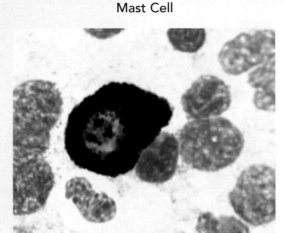

Figure 23-8 Mast cell.

DESCRIPTION: Large cell (12-25 μm) with round to oval nucleus; cytoplasm is colorless to lavender with many dark blue to black granules that may obscure the nucleus. Constitute <1% of bone marrow cells. Increased numbers may be seen in allergic inflammation and anaphylaxis.

ARTIFACTS IN PERIPHERAL BLOOD SMEARS

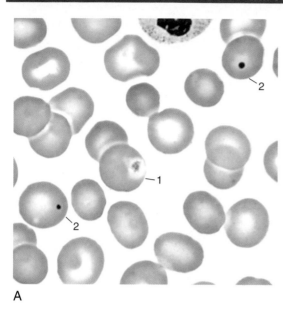

A

Figure 23-9A Platelet on RBC *(1)* or Howell–Jolly bodies *(2)* may be confused with malarial parasites (see Figure 22-1) (PB ×1000).

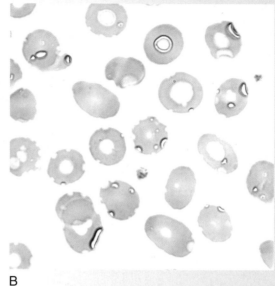

B

Figure 23-9B Water artifact may be confused with malaria (see Figure 22-1) or Cabot ring (see Figure 12-4) (PB ×1000).

Note in Figure 23-9C that precipitate is in focus, but the cells are not. If bacteria are present within a cell, both cell and bacteria should be in focus at the same time.

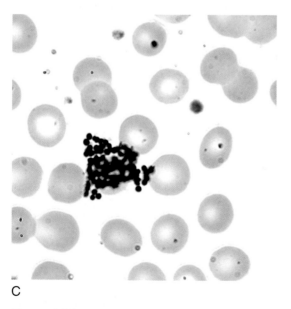

C

Figure 23-9C Precipitated stain—may be confused with bacteria (see Figure 22-6) (PB ×1000).

LEUKOCYTE ARTIFACT

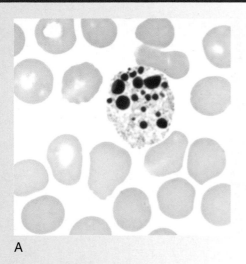

A

Figure 23-10A Pyknosis (PB ×1000).

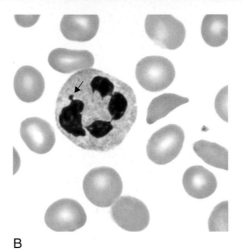

B

Figure 23-10B Barr body (PB ×1000).

DESCRIPTION: Nuclear degeneration appearing as a darkly stained structure with less mass
Associated with: Peripheral smears made from old blood; cell death

DESCRIPTION: Small, round, well-defined projection of nuclear chromatin connected to the nucleus by a strand of chromatin
SIGNIFICANCE: None

DESCRIPTION: Platelets adhering to neutrophils
Associated with: Blood collected in ethylenediaminetetraacetic acid (EDTA) in rare individuals; may cause falsely decreased platelet counts

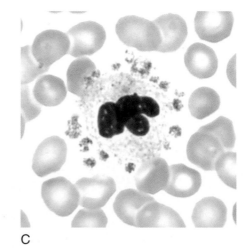

C

Figure 23-10C Platelet satellitism (PB ×1000).

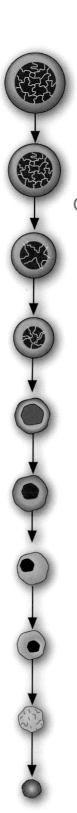

CHAPTER

24

Normal Newborn Peripheral Blood Morphology

In the normal, full-term newborn, peripheral blood collected within the first 12 hours of birth has distinctive morphology. Some morphologic changes persist for up to 3 to 5 days after birth. These changes should be recognized as physiologic and not pathologic. For a fuller discussion of hematology in the newborn, the reader is referred to a hematology textbook such as *Hematology: Clinical Principles and Applications** or a pediatric hematology text such as *Nathan and Oski's Hematology of Infancy and Childhood.*[†]

Entire books have been written to address abnormal hematology in neonates, and especially in the premature infant. This chapter will not attempt to address those disorders, but will depict morphologic changes commonly seen in the normal newborn.

Erythrocyte morphology demonstrates macrocytes, with a mean cell volume (MCV) of 110 ± 15 fL, which drops dramatically after the first 12 hours. Up to 3 to 10 orthochromic normoblasts (nucleated red blood cells [NRBCs]) may be seen per 100 white blood cells (WBCs) and should disappear by day 5. Polychromasia reflects the erythropoietic activity of the newborn. Anisocytosis is reflected in the red blood cell distribution width index (RDW), which ranges from 15.2% to 18.0%.

Occasional spherocytes are common, varying from one every two fields to one or more in every field.

Newborn total leukocyte counts are higher than adults and newborns have more polymorphonuclear and band neutrophils than at any other time in childhood.[‡] An occasional metamyelocyte may be seen without evidence of infection. Monocyte morphology is similar to that of the adult.

Lymphocyte morphology is pleomorphic, spanning the range from reactive to mature. The presence of a nucleolus in not uncommon; however, the chromatin pattern is coarse and not as fine as seen in blasts. Caution must be exercised to correctly identify blasts that may indicate a pathologic condition.

---

* Rodak BF, Fritsma GA, Doig K: *Hematology: clinical principles and applications*, ed 3, St Louis, 2007, Saunders.
[†] Nathan DG, Orkin SH, Ginsburg D, Look AT: *Nathan and Oski's hematology of infancy and childhood*, ed 6, St Louis, 2003, Saunders.
[‡] Quinn CT, Buchanan GR: Hematopoiesis and hematologic diseases. In McMillan JA, Feigin RD, DeAngelis C, Jones MD, editors: *Oski's pediatrics*, Philadelphia, 2006, Lippincott Williams and Wilkins.

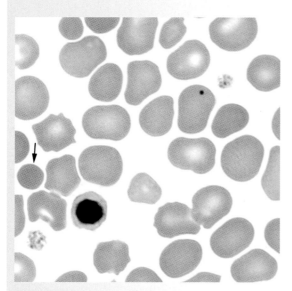

Figure 24-1 Peripheral blood from a neonate demonstrating macrocytes, polychromasia, nucleated red blood cell (NRBC), Howell-Jolly body and one spherocyte *(arrow)* (PB × 1000).

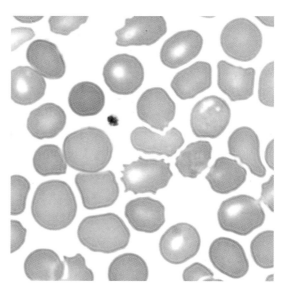

Figure 24-2 Peripheral blood from a normal neonate demonstrating polychromasia, anisocytosis, echinocytes, and spherocytes (PB × 1000).

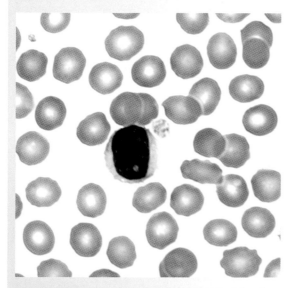

Figure 24-3 Lymphocyte from neonate blood. Although there appears to be a nucleolus, the chromatin pattern is coarse (PB × 1000).

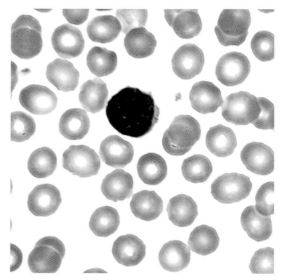

Figure 24-4 Lymphocyte from a normal neonate (PB × 1000).

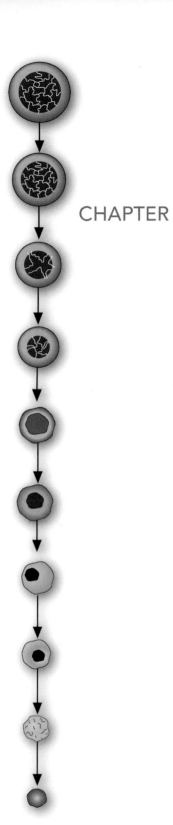

25

Body Fluids

Fluid in the cavities that surround organs may serve as a lubricant or shock absorber, provide circulation of nutrients, or function for collection of waste. Evaluation of body fluids may include total volume, gross appearance, total cell count, differential cell count, identification of crystals, biochemical analysis, microbiological examination, immunological studies, and cytological examination. The most common body fluid specimens received in the laboratory are cerebrospinal fluid (CSF); pleural, peritoneal, and pericardial fluids (together known as *serous fluids*); and synovial fluids. Under normal circumstances the only fluid that is present in an amount large enough to sample is CSF. Therefore, when other fluids are present in detectable amounts, disease is suspected.

This atlas addresses primarily the elements of fluids that are observable through a microscope. For a more detailed explanation of body fluids, the reader should consult a hematology or urinalysis textbook that includes a discussion of body fluids, such as *Hematology: Clinical Principles and Applications** or *Fundamentals of Urine and Body Fluid Analysis*.[†]

Because the number of cells in fluids is often very small, a concentrated specimen is preferable for performing the morphological examination. Preparation of slides using a cytocentrifuge is the method commonly used. This centrifuge spins at a low rate of speed in order to minimize distortion of cells, concentrating the cells into a "button" on a small area of the glass slide. The three elements of the cytocentrifuge are a cytofunnel, filter paper to absorb excess fluid, and a glass slide. These elements are clipped together in a clip assembly, and the entire apparatus is then centrifuged slowly. Excess fluid is absorbed by the filter paper, leaving a monolayer of cells in a small button on the slide. When the cytospin slide is removed from the centrifuge, it should be dry. If the cell button is still wet, the centrifugation time may need to be extended.

When preparing cytocentrifuge slides, a consistent amount of fluid should be used to generate a consistent yield of cells. Usually two to six drops of fluid are used depending on the nucleated cell count. Five drops of fluid will generally yield enough cells to perform a 100-cell differential if the nucleated cell count is at least $3/mm^3$. For very high counts, a dilution with normal saline may be made. The area of the slide where the cell button will be deposited should be marked with a wax pencil in case the number of cells recovered is small and difficult to locate. Alternatively, specially marked slides can be used (Figure 25-1).

There may be some distortion of cells as a result of centrifugation, or when cell counts are high. In order to minimize distortion when nucleated cell counts are high, dilutions with normal saline should be made before centrifugation. When the red blood cell count is extremely high (more than 1 million), the slide should be made in the same manner as the peripheral blood smear slide (see Chapter 1). However, the examination of the smear should be performed at the end of the slide rather than the battlement pattern used

---

* Rodak BF, Fritsma GA, Doig K: *Hematology: clinical principles and applications*, ed 3, St Louis, 2007, Saunders.
[†] Brunzel NA: *Fundamentals of urine and body fluid analysis*, ed 2, St Louis, 2004, Saunders.

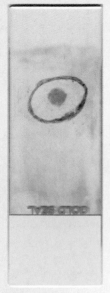

A

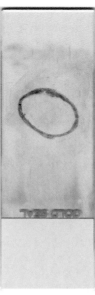

B

Figure 25-1A Wright-stained cytocentrifuge slide demonstrating a concentrated button of cells within the marked circle.

Figure 25-1B Wright-stained cytocentrifuge slide from a cerebrospinal fluid containing very few cells, demonstrating the importance of marking the cell concentration area.

for blood smears. This is because the larger, and usually more significant cells, are likely to be pushed to the end of the slide.

When examining the cytospin slide, the entire cell button should be scanned under the 10 × objective to search for the presence of tumor cells. The 50 × or 100 × oil immersion lens should be used to differentiate the white blood cells. For the performance of the differential, any area of the cell button may be used, but if the cell count is low, a systematic pattern starting at one end of the side of the button and working toward the other is recommended.

Any cell that is seen in the peripheral blood may be found in a body fluid in addition to cells specific to that fluid (e.g., cells lining the organ space, such as mesothelial cells, macrophages, tumor cells). However, the cells look somewhat different than in peripheral blood and some in vivo degeneration is normal. The presence of organisms, such as yeast and bacteria, should also be noted (see Figures 25-12 to 25-14).

CELLS COMMONLY SEEN IN CEREBROSPINAL FLUID

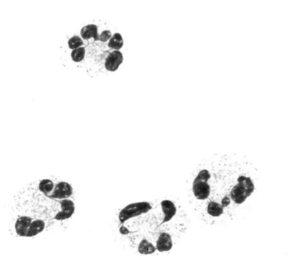

Figure 25-2 Polymorphonuclear neutrophils (PMNs) (CSF ×1000).

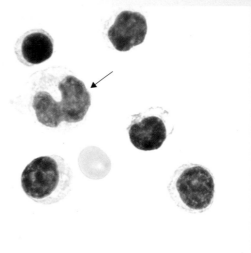

Figure 25-3 Lymphocytes and monocyte *(arrow)* (CSF ×1000).

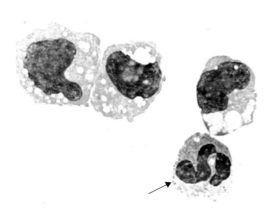

Figure 25-4 Monocytes and polymorphonuclear neutrophil *(arrow)* (CSF ×1000).

COMMENTS: Small numbers of polymorphonuclear neutrophils (PMNs), lymphocytes, and monocytes may be seen in normal cerebrospinal fluid.

Increased numbers of PMNs are associated with bacterial meningitis; early stages of viral, fungal, and tubercular meningitis; intracranial hemorrhage; intrathecal injections; central nervous system (CNS) infarct; malignancy; or abscess.

Increased number of lymphocytes and monocytes are associated with viral, fungal, tubercular and bacterial meningitis, and multiple sclerosis.

NOTE: These cells may be the only class of cell in the specimen, but are often found as a mixture of lymphocytes and monocytes and PMNs.

CELLS SOMETIMES FOUND IN CEREBROSPINAL FLUID

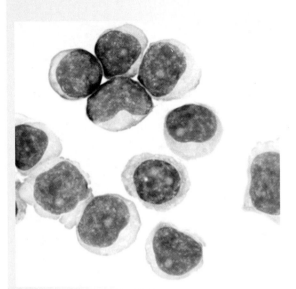

Figure 25-5 Reactive lymphocytes (CSF ×1000).

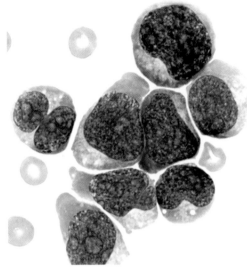

Figure 25-6 Acute lymphoid leukemia (ALL) blasts (CSF ×1000).

Reactive lymphocytes (Figure 25-5) are associated with viral meningitis and other antigenic stimulation. As a result of pleomorphism, the cells will vary in size; nuclear shape may be irregular and cytoplasm may be scant to abundant with pale to intense staining characteristics. (See description of reactive lymphocytes, Figure 15-13.)

Blasts in the CSF may have some of the characteristics of the acute lymphoid leukemia (ALL) blasts seen in the peripheral blood (Figure 25-6; see Chapter 17). It is not unusual for ALL to have central nervous system (CNS) involvement and blasts may be present in the CSF before being observed in the peripheral blood.

NOTE: Blasts have less heterogeneity in size and staining characteristics than reactive lymphocytes.

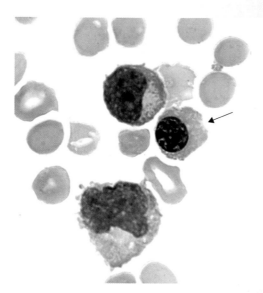

Figure 25-7 Nucleated red blood cells
(CSF ×1000).

Associated with: Traumatic lumbar tap in premature infants, blood dyscrasias with circulating NRBCs, and bone marrow contamination of CSF.

CELLS SOMETIMES FOUND IN CEREBROSPINAL FLUID AFTER CENTRAL NERVOUS SYSTEM HEMORRHAGE

The following sequence of events is a typical reaction to intracranial hemorrhage or repeated lumbar punctures:

1. PMNs and macrophages—appear within 2 to 4 hours
2. Erythrophages—identifiable from 1 to 7 days
3. Siderophages—observable from 2 days to 2 months
4. Hematoidin crystals—recognizable in 2 to 4 weeks

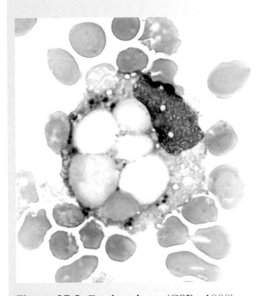

Figure 25-8 Erythrophage (CSF ×1000).

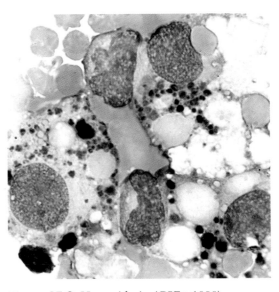

Figure 25-9 Hemosiderin (CSF ×1000).

A macrophage with engulfed red blood cells (RBCs) is shown in Figure 25-8. RBCs are digested by enzymatic activity within the macrophage. The digestion process causes the RBCs to lose color and to appear as vacuoles within the cytoplasm of some macrophages.

Blue to black granules containing iron, resulting from the degradation of hemoglobin, may be present in CSF for up to 8 weeks after intracranial hemorrhage. The cellular inclusions can be positively identified with an iron stain (Figure 25-9).

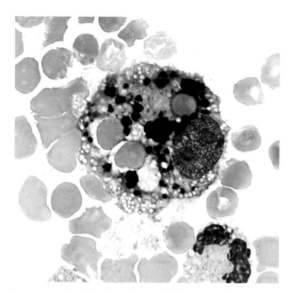

Figure 25-10 Siderophage (CSF ×1000).

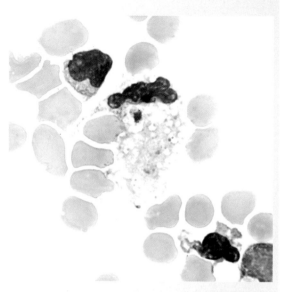

Figure 25-11 Hematoidin within macrophage (CSF ×1000).

Macrophage containing hemosiderin.

Gold intracellular crystals composed of bilirubin. Hematoidin is the result of the catabolism of hemoglobin and may be present for several weeks after CNS hemorrhage.

NOTE: Macrophages may display the presence of a variety of particles within one cell. For example, one macrophage may contain hemosiderin and hematoidin.

ORGANISMS SOMETIMES FOUND IN CEREBROSPINAL FLUID

Cerebrospinal fluid is a sterile body fluid. The following are examples of some organisms that have been seen in CSF, but it is far from an all-inclusive list of possibilities. Note that organisms may be seen intracellular, extracellular, or both.

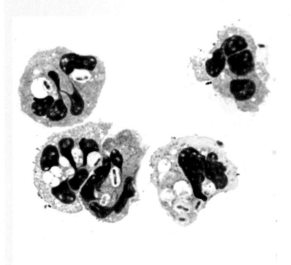

Figure 25-12 Bacteria engulfed by neutrophils (CSF ×1000).

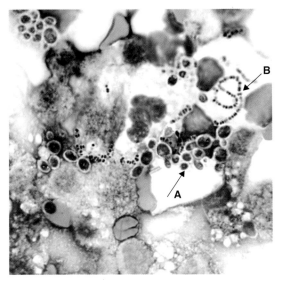

Figure 25-13 *Histoplasma capsulatum (A)* within macrophage (CSF ×1000). Note the presence of bacteria in chains *(B)*.

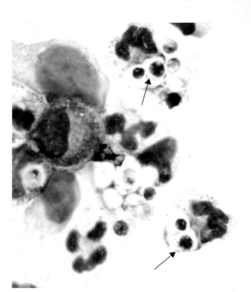

Figure 25-14 *Cryptococcus neoformans* inside neutrophil (CSF ×1000).

BLOOD CELLS SOMETIMES FOUND IN SEROUS BODY FLUIDS (PLEURAL, PERICARDIAL, AND PERITONEAL)

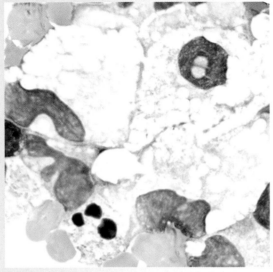

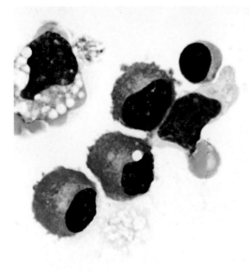

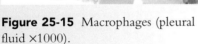

Figure 25-15 Macrophages (pleural fluid ×1000).

Figure 25-16 Plasma cells (pleural fluid ×1000).

DESCRIPTION: Large cells with eccentric nuclei and vacuolated cytoplasm. May be seen with or without inclusions, such as RBCs, siderotic granules, or lipids.

Associated with: Rheumatoid arthritis, malignancy, tuberculosis, and other conditions that exhibit lymphocytosis

NOTE: Any of the cell types found in the peripheral blood may be found in serous fluids.

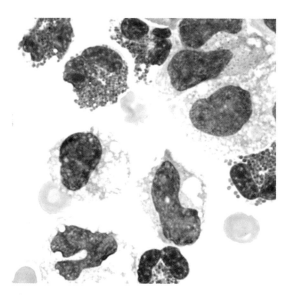

Figure 25-17 Eosinophils (pleural fluid ×1000).

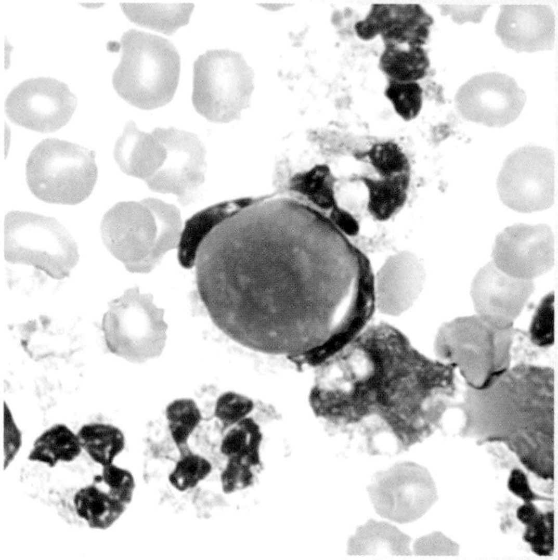

Figure 25-18 Lupus erythematosus (LE) cell (pleural fluid ×1000).

Associated with: Allergy, air, and/or foreign matter within the body cavity, parasites

Intact neutrophil with engulfed homogenous mass. The mass displaces the nucleus of the neutrophil and is composed of degenerated nuclear material. Lupus erythematosus (LE) cells are formed in vivo and in vitro in serous fluids. LE cells may also form in synovial fluids.

Associated with: Lupus erythematosus

MESOTHELIAL CELLS

Mesothelial cells are shed from membranes lining body cavities and are often found in serous fluids.

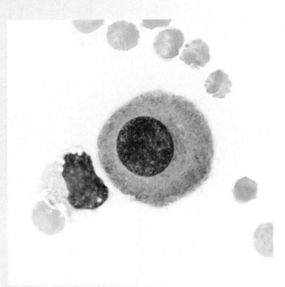

Figure 25-19 Mesothelial cell with pale blue cytoplasm (pleural fluid ×1000).

Figure 25-20 Mesothelial cells with deeply basophilic cytoplasm (pleural fluid ×1000).

SHAPE: Pleomorphic
SIZE: 12-30 µm
NUCLEUS: Round to oval with smooth nuclear borders. Nucleus may be eccentric or multinucleated, making the distinction between the mesothelial and plasma cell difficult.
NUCLEOLI: 1-3, uniform in size and shape
CHROMATIN: Fine, evenly distributed
CYTOPLASM: Abundant, light gray to deeply basophilic
VACUOLES: Occasionally

NOTE: Mesothelial cells may appear as single cells in clumps or sheets. The clumping of cells to one another and the variability of appearance require careful observation to accurately differentiate mesothelial cells from malignant cells. Three characteristics can aid in this determination:

1. Mesothelial cells on a smear tend to be similar to one another.
2. The nuclear membrane appears smooth by light microscopy.
3. Mesothelial cells maintain cytoplasmic borders. When appearing in clumps, there may be clear spaces between the cells. These are often referred to as "windows."

MULTINUCLEATED MESOTHELIAL CELLS

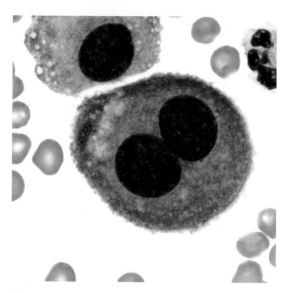

Figure 25-21 Binucleated mesothelial cell (pleural fluid ×1000).

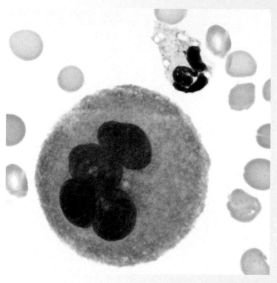

Figure 25-22 Multinucleated mesothelial cell (pleural fluid ×1000).

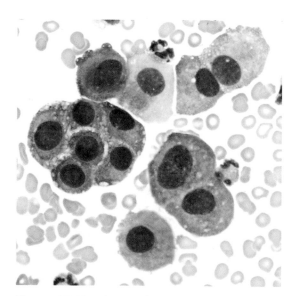

Figure 25-23 Clump of mesothelial cells. Note "windows" in the large clump (pleural fluid ×500).

It is not always possible to distinguish malignant cells from mesothelial cells with the sole use of the light microscope. The following criteria for malignant cells may aid in this distinction:

NUCLEUS: High N:C ratio, membrane irregular
NUCLEOLI: Multiple, large with irregular staining
CHROMATIN: Hyperchromatic with uneven distribution
CYTOPLASM: Irregular membrane

Cells tend to form clumps with cytoplasmic molding. The boundaries between cells may be indistinguishable.

NOTE: Smears with cells displaying one or more of the above characteristics should be referred to a qualified cytologist for confirmation. See Table 25-1 for a comparison of benign and malignant features.

TABLE 25-1 Characteristics of Benign and Malignant Cells

Benign	Malignant
Occasional large cells	Many cells may be very large
Light to dark staining	May be very basophilic
Rare mitotic figures	May have several mitotic figures
Round to oval nucleus; nuclei are uniform size with varying amounts of cytoplasm	May have irregular or bizarre nuclear shape
Smooth nuclear edge	Edges of nucleus may be indistinct and irregular
Nucleus intact	Nucleus may be disintegrated at edges
Nucleoli are small, if present	Nucleoli may be large and prominent
In multinuclear cells (mesothelial), all nuclei have similar appearance (size and shape)	Multinuclear cells have varying sizes and shapes of nuclei
Moderate to small N:C ratio	May have high N:C ratio
Clumps of cells have similar appearance among cells, are on the same plane of focus, and may have "windows" between cells	Clumps of cells contain cells of varying sizes and shapes, are "three-dimensional" (have to focus up and down to see all cells), and have dark-staining borders; no "windows" between cells

From Rodak BF, Fritsma GA, Doig K: *Hematology: clinical principles and applications*, ed 3, St Louis, 2007, Saunders.
N:C, Nuclear:cytoplasmic.

MALIGNANT CELLS SOMETIMES SEEN IN SEROUS FLUIDS

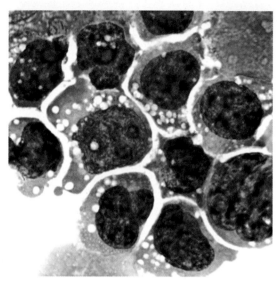

Figure 25-24   Non-Hodgkin lymphoma (pleural fluid ×1000).

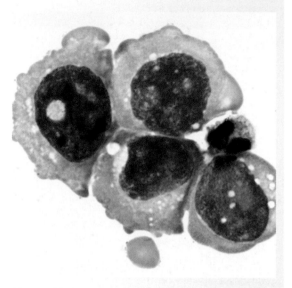

Figure 25-25   Breast tumor metastases (pleural fluid ×1000).

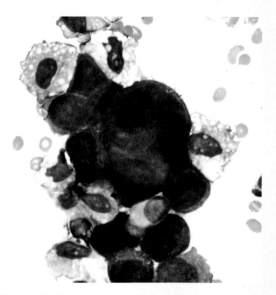

Figure 25-26   Malignant tumor (pleural fluid ×500). Note molding of cytoplasm (no "windows" between cells).

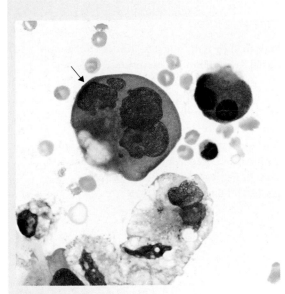

Figure 25-27 Adenocarcinoma, metastases from uterine cancer (pleural fluid ×500). Note irregular nuclear membranes.

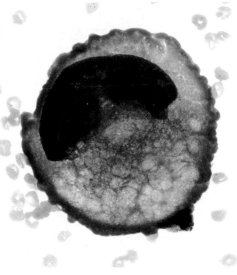

Figure 25-28 Malignant tumor (pleural fluid ×500).

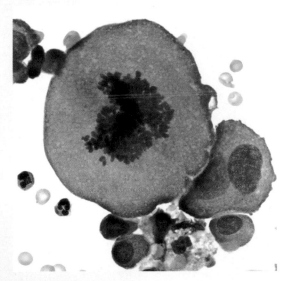

Figure 25-29 Mitotic figure in malignancy (pleural fluid ×500).

Mitotic figures may be found in normal fluids and are not necessarily an indication of malignancy. The size of this mitotic figure, however, is quite large, and malignant cells were easily found.

CRYSTALS SOMETIMES FOUND IN SYNOVIAL FLUID

Cells that may be found in normal synovial fluids include lymphocytes, monocytes, and synovial cells. Synovial cells, which line the synovial cavity, resemble mesothelial cells (see Figure 25-19) but are smaller and less numerous. Increased numbers of polymorphonuclear neutrophils may be seen in bacterial infection and acute inflammation. When neutrophils are seen, a careful search for bacteria should be performed. Tumor cells are possible but quite rare. LE cells may also be seen (see Figure 25-18).

It is important to perform a careful evaluation for crystals in synovial fluid. Although it is not necessary to use a stain, Wright stain is sometimes used. A polarizing microscope with a red compensator should always be used for confirmation. The most common crystals are monosodium urate, calcium pyrophosphate, and cholesterol.

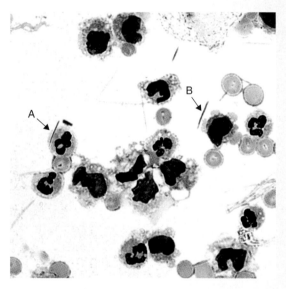

Figure 25-30 Monosodium urate crystals (synovial fluid ×1000) (Wright stain).

Figure 25-30 shows needlelike crystals with pointed ends, which may be intracellular *(A)*, extracellular *(B)*, or both.

Associated with: Gout

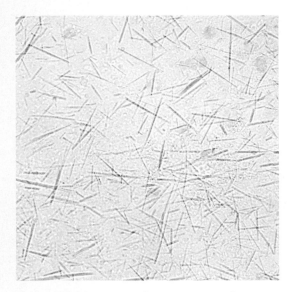

Figure 25-31 Monosodium urate crystals (synovial fluid ×1000) (unstained). (Courtesy George Girgis, MT [ASCP], Indiana University Medical Center.)

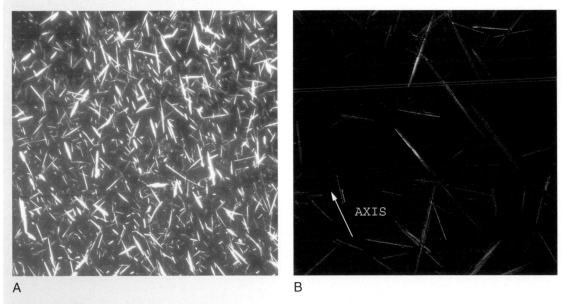

A   B

Figure 25-32 Monosodium urate crystals, polarized light microscopy **(A)** and with red compensator **(B)** (synovial fluid ×1000). (Courtesy George Girgis, MT [ASCP], Indiana University Medical Center.)

Note the orientation of the crystals and corresponding colors. Crystals appear yellow when parallel to the axis of the compensator; blue when perpendicular to the axis (negative birefringence).

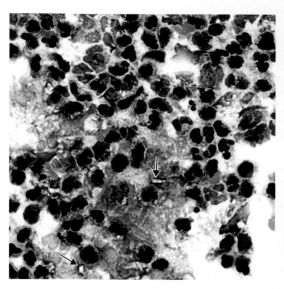

Figure 25-33 Calcium pyrophosphate crystals (synovial fluid ×1000) (Wright stain).

Rhomboid, rodlike chunky crystals—may be intracellular, extracellular, or both

Associated with: Pseudogout or pyrophosphate gout

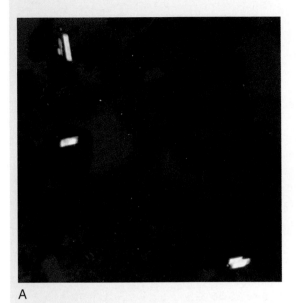

A

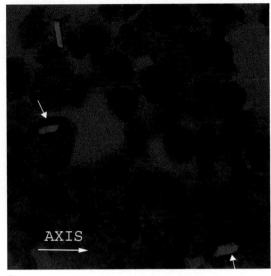

B

Figure 25-34A Calcium pyrophosphate crystals, polarized light microscopy (synovial fluid ×1000). (Courtesy George Girgis, MT [ASCP], Indiana University Medical Center.)

Figure 25-34B Calcium pyrophosphate crystals, polarized with red compensator (synovial fluid ×1000). (Courtesy George Girgis, MT [ASCP], Indiana University Medical Center.)

Note the orientation of the crystals and corresponding colors. Crystals appear blue when parallel to the axis of the compensator or yellow when perpendicular to the axis (positive birefringence). Calcium pyrophosphate is only weakly birefringent, so that the colors are not as bright as monosodium urate crystals (see Figure 25-32).

Figure 25-35 Cholesterol crystals (synovial fluid ×500).

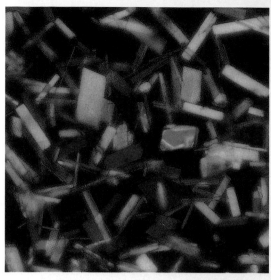

Figure 25-36 Cholesterol crystals (synovial fluid ×500) (polarized light microscopy). (Courtesy George Girgis, MT [ASCP], Indiana University Medical Center.)

Large, flat rectangular plates with notched corners.

Associated with: Chronic inflammatory conditions and considered a nonspecific finding

It is necessary to use polarized light for confirmation of cholesterol crystals, but it is not necessary to use a red compensator.

OTHER STRUCTURES SOMETIMES SEEN IN BODY FLUIDS

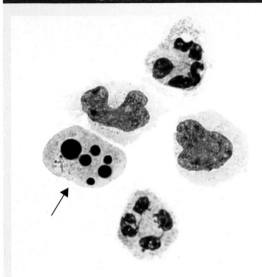

Figure 25-37 Pyknosis (pleural fluid ×500).

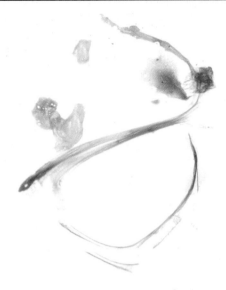

Figure 25-38 Artifact (pleural fluid ×500).

Intracellular nuclear degeneration appearing as darkly stained mass(es) (Figure 25-37, *arrow*), compared to two normal polymorphonuclear cells. Contrary to pyknosis seen in peripheral blood, pyknotic figures in body fluids can develop in vivo.

Fibers from the filter paper may appear near the edges of the slide. Fibers may be birefringent, but lack the sharp pointed ends of monosodium urate crystals.

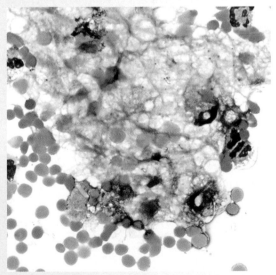

Figure 25-39 Brain tissue (CSF ×500).

The specimen in Figure 25-39 is from a patient who experienced head trauma.

Index

Page numbers followed by *b* indicate boxes; *t,* tables.